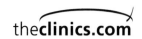

CLINICS IN PODIATRIC MEDICINE AND SURGERY OF NORTH AMERICA

Pediatric Foot and Ankle Disorders

GUEST EDITOR
Jonathan M. Labovitz, DPM

CONSULTING EDITOR
Vincent J. Mandracchia, DPM, MS

January 2006 • Volume 23 • Number 1

SAUNDERS

An Imprint of Elsevier, Inc.
PHILADELPHIA   LONDON   TORONTO   MONTREAL   SYDNEY   TOKYO

W.B. SAUNDERS COMPANY
A Division of Elsevier Inc.

1600 John F. Kennedy Blvd., Suite 1800, Philadelphia, PA 19103-2899

http://www.theclinics.com

CLINICS IN PODIATRIC MEDICINE
AND SURGERY   Volume 23, Number 1
January 2006   ISSN 0891-8422
Editor: Karen Sorensen   ISBN 1-4160-3379-3

Reprints. For copies of 100 or more of articles in this publication, please contact the Commercial Reprints Department, Elsevier Inc., 360 Park Avenue South, New York, New York 10010-1710 Tel.: (212) 633-3813, Fax: (212) 462-1935, e-mail: reprints@elsevier.com

Clinics in Podiatric Medicine and Surgery (ISSN 0891-8422) is published quarterly by Elsevier. Corporate and editorial Offices: 1600 John F. Kennedy Blvd., Suite 1800, Philadelphia, PA 19103-2899. Accounting and circulation offices: 6277 Sea Harbor Drive, Orlando, FL 32887–4800. Periodicals postage paid at Orlando, FL 32862, and additional mailing offices. Subscription prices are $175.00 per year for US individuals, $280.00 per year for US institutions, $90.00 per year for US students and residents, $210.00 per year for Canadian individuals, $340.00 per year for Canadian institutions, $235.00 for international individuals, $340.00 for international institutions and $120.00 per year for Canadian and foreign students/residents. To receive student/resident rate, orders must be accompanied by name of affiliated institution, date of term, and the *signature* of program/residency coordinator on institution letterhead. Orders will be billed at individual rate until proof of status is received. Foreign air speed delivery is included in all *Clinics* subscription prices. All prices are subject to change without notice. POSTMASTER: Send address changes to *Clinics in Podiatric Medicine and Surgery*, W.B. Saunders Company, Periodicals Fulfillment, Orlando, FL 32887-4800. **Customer Service: 1-800-654-2452 (US). From outside of the US, call 1-407-345-1000.**

Clinics in Podiatric Medicine and Surgery is covered in *Index Medicus* and *EMBASE/ Excerpta Medica.*

Printed in the United States of America.

CONSULTING EDITOR

VINCENT J. MANDRACCHIA, DPM, MS, Section Chief, Podiatric Surgery, Department of Surgery, Broadlawns Medical Center; and Clinical Professor, Department of Podiatric Medicine and Surgery, College of Podiatric Medicine and Surgery, Des Moines University–Osteopathic Medicine Center, Des Moines, Iowa

GUEST EDITOR

JONATHAN M. LABOVITZ, DPM, Fellow, American College of Foot and Ankle Surgeons; Private Practice, West Torrance Podiatrists Group, Inc.; Attending Staff, West Los Angeles Veterans Affairs Medical Center, Los Angeles, California; Faculty, Baja Project for Crippled Children, Incorporated

CONTRIBUTORS

MARC A. BENARD, DPM, FACFAOM, FACFAS, Diplomate of the American Board of Podiatric Orthopedics and Primary Podiatric Medicine and the American Board of Podiatric Surgery; Private Practice, Torrance, California; Co-Director, Baja Project for Crippled Children, Incorporated

MARK D. DOLLARD, DPM, Fellow, American College of Foot and Ankle Surgeons; Fellow, American Academy of Podiatric Sports Medicine; Past National Chairman, 1994–1996, Sports Medicine Committee, USA Amateur Athletic Union; Clinical Instructor, Inova Podiatric Surgical Residency Program, Inova Fairfax Hospital, Fairfax, Virginia; Clinical Instructor, Department of Orthopedics, Georgetown University Medical Center, Washington, DC; Private Practice, Loudoun Foot and Ankle Center, Sterling, Virginia

IAN J. GALLEY, MD, Fellow, Rubin Institute for Advanced Orthopedics, Sinai Hospital of Baltimore, Baltimore, Maryland

WOLFGANG GRECHENIG, MD, Associate Professor of Orthopedic Trauma, Department of Trauma, Medical University Graz, Graz, Austria

NICHOLAS A. GRUMBINE, DPM, Fellow, American College of Foot and Ankle Surgeons; Private Practice, Orange, California; Senior Attending, Baja Project for Crippled Children, Incorporated

ROBERT HALLIVIS, DPM, Fellow, American College of Foot and Ankle Surgeons; Adjunct Clinical Assistant Professor, Department of Podiatric Medicine, Temple University School of Podiatric Medicine; Residency Training Committee, Podiatric Residency Program, Inova Fairfax Hospital, Fairfax, Virginia; Private Practice, Dominion Foot and Ankle Consultants PC, Annandale, Virginia

RANDOLF HAMMERL, MD, Consultant of Internal Medicine, Department of Internal Medicine, Federal Hospital Fuerstenfeld, Styria, Austria

EDWIN J. HARRIS, DPM, FACFAS, Diplomate of the American Board of Podiatric Surgery and the American Board of Podiatric Orthopedics and Primary Podiatric Medicine; Associate Clinical Professor of Orthopaedics and Rehabilitation, Department of Orthopaedic Surgery, Stritch School of Medicine, Loyola University Medical Center, Maywood, Illinois; Faculty, Dr. William M. Scholl College of Podiatric Medicine, Rosalind Franklin University of Health Sciences; Private Practice in Pediatric Podiatry, Philadelphia, Pennsylvania

JOHN E. HERZENBERG, MD, FRCSC, Rubin Institute for Advanced Orthopedics, Chief, Pediatric Orthopedics, Sinai Hospital of Baltimore, Baltimore, Maryland; Co-Director, International Center for Limb Lengthening

JONATHAN M. LABOVITZ, DPM, Fellow, American College of Foot and Ankle Surgeons; Private Practice, West Torrance Podiatrists Group, Inc.; Attending Staff, West Los Angeles Veterans Affairs Medical Center, Los Angeles, California; Faculty, Baja Project for Crippled Children, Incorporated

BRADLEY M. LAMM, DPM, Head, Podiatry Section, Rubin Institute for Advanced Orthopedics, Sinai Hospital of Baltimore, Baltimore, Maryland

JOHANNES MAYR, MD, Professor of Pediatric Surgery, Department of Pediatric Surgery, University Children's Hospital, Basel, Switzerland

DROR PALEY, MD, FRCSC, Director, Rubin Institute for Advanced Orthopedics, Sinai Hospital of Baltimore, Baltimore, Maryland; Co-Director, International Center for Limb Lengthening

GEROLF PEICHA, MD, Associate Professor of Orthopedic Trauma, Department of Trauma, Medical University Graz, Graz, Austria

DAVID PONTELL, DPM, Fellow, American College of Foot and Ankle Surgeons; Adjunct Clinical Assistant Professor, Department of Podiatric Medicine, Temple University School of Podiatric Medicine; Residency Training Committee, Podiatric Residency Program, Inova Fairfax Hospital, Fairfax, Virginia; Private Practice, Dominion Foot and Ankle Consultants PC, Annandale, Virginia

HAROLD D. SCHOENHAUS, DPM, FACFAOM, FACFAS, Diplomate of the American Board of Podiatric Orthopedics and Primary Podiatric Medicine and the American Board of Podiatric Surgery; Professor of Orthopedics, Temple University School of Podiatric Medicine, Philadelphia, Pennsylvania

JARROD M. SHAPIRO, DPM, Chief Podiatric Resident, Department of Podiatry, Botsford General Hospital, Farmington Hills, Michigan

STEPHEN SILVANI, DPM, Fellow, American College of Foot and Ankle Surgeons; Diplomate, American Board of Podiatric Surgeons; Orthopedic Department, Walnut Creek, California; Attending Staff, The San Francisco Bay Area Foot and Ankle Residency Program; Fellow and Past President of the American College of Foot and Ankle Pediatrics; Podiatric Advisor, Northwest Podiatric Foundation; President, Board of Directors, American Board of Podiatric Surgery

ERICH SORANTIN, MD, Associate Professor of Radiology, Division of Pediatric Radiology, Medical University Graz, Graz, Austria

SHAWN C. STANDARD, MD, Pediatric Orthopedic Surgeon, Rubin Institute for Advanced Orthopedics, Sinai Hospital of Baltimore, Baltimore, Maryland

STEPHEN C. WAN, DPM, Fellow, American College of Foot and Ankle Surgeons; Attending Staff, Los Angeles County–University of Southern California Medical Center, Los Angeles, California

ANDREAS WEIGLEIN, MD, Associate Professor of Anatomy, Institute of Anatomy, Medical University Graz, Graz, Austria

JEFFREY Y. YUNG, DPM, FACFAS, Faculty, Residency Training Committee, Botsford General Hospital, Farmington Hills, Michigan; Assistant Clinical Professor, Michigan State University; Faculty, Baja Project for Crippled Children, Incorporated

CONTENTS

> The pediatric foot and ankle examination is a specialized yet important skill for the modern podiatric medical practitioner. An organized and sequential history and physical examination yields a thorough database of information for which to establish a successful treatment regimen.

> Metatarsus adductus deformity should be recognized and addressed appropriately and in a timely fashion so as to achieve an effective correction with low rates of recurrence. Early diagnosis and treatment are of paramount importance, because spontaneous resolution is rare. Although nonoperative treatment is desirable via manipulation and soft tissue stretching and serial cast immobilization, appropriate surgical intervention needs to be used on occasion to achieve correction of resistant cases. Depending on the severity and flexibility of the deformity and the age of the patient, various methods of surgical reconstruction are available. A long-standing untreated or undertreated adductus deformity can lead to the formation of a skewfoot deformity with more significant symptoms and deformity. Treatment of this deformity is rarely successful by nonoperative

means, and appropriate surgical procedures addressing the metatarsal adductus component and the flatfoot component can be used for correction of the dysfunctional or symptomatic skewfoot.

The talar neck osteotomy is done at the junction of the head and neck of the talus, frequently in conjunction with desmoplasty and posterior tibial tendon advancement. This is done effectively to correct severe deformities involving the talus. The correction produces a structural realignment of the talar head. Adjunctive procedures are also done when these are deformities involving the posterior column, lateral column, and/or medial column. A 27-year follow-up study is presented containing data from 215 procedures on 117 patients with a minimum of one year follow-up.

The author presents an alternative approach to the pediatric flexible pes planovalgus patient. Hopefully, this algorithm can serve as a guide and not as a rule. It is meant to serve the foot and ankle surgeon as a means of eliminating the arbitrary assignment of a flatfoot to procedures. Instead, the algorithm assigns procedures to a type of flatfoot. The specific procedures listed are a guide to reduce our failures while continually improving our successes.

Pediatric clinical management is highly specialized. Problems are complex and often complicated by other medical issues that dictate limitations on therapeutic options. Appropriate diagnosis and successful clinical management depend on the experience and skill of the surgeon. This roundtable discussion focuses on seven difficult cases and presents the views of three experienced and skilled experts in the field.

Traditional treatment for clubfoot usually includes initial casting and an extensive posterior medial soft tissue release with biplanar pinning, followed by more casting. This treatment has significant risks, complications, and the potential for a poorer prognosis as the patients age, usually with stiff and scarred feet. In contradistinction, Ignacio Ponseti has been using his unique technique of clubfoot manipulation, casting, and Achilles tenotomy for more than 50 years with a high degree of success. Currently, there are many peer-reviewed and independently verified studies that replicate his success in treating clubfoot. This technique is easy to learn and is becoming the accepted treatment of idiopathic clubfoot all over the world.

During the last decade, external fixation for the pediatric foot and ankle has evolved as a result of advances in technology (eg, Taylor spatial frame, hydroxyapatite-coated external fixator pins) and preoperative deformity planning. Although complications are common, most are minor and can be addressed nonoperatively while treatment continues. This article reviews the indications and applications of external fixation for soft tissue contractures, idiopathic and teratologic clubfoot, osteotomies, metatarsal lengthening, tibial lengthening, and foot and ankle trauma.

The challenge of managing pediatric foot injuries is the identification of the rare injuries that require operative treatment and the management of complications such as compartment syndrome, post-traumatic foot deformities, and avascular necrosis. With these complications in mind, the authors discuss fractures of the talus, calcaneus, lesser tarsal bones, Lisfranc's joint, metarsals, and phalanges. Dislocation of metatarsophalangeal or interphalangeal joints is also discussed.

Preseason preconditioning can be accomplished well over a 4-week period with a mandatory period of rest as we have discussed. Athletic participation must be guided by a gradual increase of skills performance in the child assessed after a responsible preconditioning program applying physiologic parameters as outlined. Clearly, designing a preconditioning program is a dynamic process when accounting for all the variables in training discussed so far. Despite the physiologic demands of sport and training, we still need to acknowledge the psychologic maturity and welfare of the child so as to ensure that the sport environment is a wholesome and emotionally rewarding experience.

Care of the youth athlete requires knowledge of developmental anatomy and specific injury patterns, which are acute or chronic in nature. We may expect that the incidence of overuse and acute foot and ankle injuries in this population is likely to increase in proportion to the number and intensity of competitive youth teams with demanding training schedules. We, as physicians, must exercise our best judgment in regard to recognizing these patterns early and instituting appropriate treatments. Return to play decisions should be based on objective criteria when available and always keeping the best interest of the athlete's future health in the forefront of our minds.

FORTHCOMING ISSUES

RECENT ISSUES

ELSEVIER
SAUNDERS

Clin Podiatr Med Surg
23 (2006) xiii–xiv

CLINICS IN
PODIATRIC
MEDICINE AND
SURGERY

Foreword

What a Novel Idea!

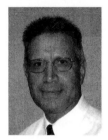

Vincent J. Mandracchia, DPM, MS
Consulting Editor

> If I had thought about it, I wouldn't have done the experiment. The literature was full of examples that said you can't do this.
>
> —Spencer Silver, on the work that led to 3M's Post-It notepads

> *Jefe:* We have stuffed many piñatas for your birthday celebration!
> *El Guapo:* How many piñatas?
> *Jefe:* Many piñatas, many!
> *El Guapo:* Jefe, would you say I have a plethora of piñatas?
> *Jefe:* Yes, El Guapo. You have a plethora.
> *El Guapo:* Jefe, what is a plethora?
>
> —*The Three Amigos* (1986)

It's not a new idea, by any means, but an idea that needs to be revisited. Multiple adjunct professorships can only serve to better the educational experience of our podiatric medical students. After all, why limit the exposure of the medical students to the faculty at the medical schools when there is a plethora of knowledge just outside the "hallowed halls?"

Private practice podiatrists have a tremendous wealth of experience-based knowledge and a rich supply of diverse pathology in their respective offices, which can only serve to enhance and augment the educational experience of our

doi:10.1016/j.cpm.2005.10.012

students. The plan is simple: incorporate all of the available sources so that the graduating podiatric medical students are not only exposed to the "wholeness" of the profession but are "fired up" and excited about their chosen profession.

The new buzzword in the world of fitness is "core" exercise. We are constantly reminded that to achieve our goals we must first concentrate on waking and developing our core. The benefit of this is to develop balance. Our colleges supply this core with their full-time dedicated faculty; however, the educational process should not be limited to the development of the core. It is essential to the survival and future development and advancement of our profession that we allow our students the ability to develop much more. This "axial" development, if you will, strengthens the core and can only come from repeated exposure to what the outside private practitioners offer, their experiences, and their patient load.

So—how to accomplish this task? It's very easy and straightforward: offer the outside practitioners in close proximity to the colleges a faculty appointment. Adjunct or clinical professorships benefit the colleges, the private practitioner, and most importantly, the students and the future of our profession. Besides, everybody likes to have a title, certainly an academic title that would impress patients—and a nice plaque for the office wall wouldn't hurt!

The addition of part-time clinical faculty only serves to strengthen the core faculty who are often overstretched in their efforts to equalize the educational experiences of the students. It also serves to strengthen the limited resources often found at the colleges. After all, in numbers there is strength.

Regardless of what "experiences" we had during our education or how much we may feel that the colleges may or may not be putting out too many students, we cannot and should not hold that against the students; none of what is occurring around them is their doing. Our only purpose is to ensure that those of us, who have the ability to do so, contribute to producing the finest podiatric medical students possible and continue the tradition of podiatry as the premier lower extremity specialist bar none.

I challenge the colleges, if they have not already done so, to include the private practitioners as clinical appointed faculty. There are a significant number of these individuals willing and able to contribute to the education of the podiatric medical students. It's a win–win situation. We certainly don't want our students to have a Napoleon Dynamite experience:

> *Grandma:* How was school?
> *Napoleon Dynamite:* The worst day of my life, what do you think?

—*Napoleon Dynamite* (2004)

Vincent J. Mandracchia, DPM, MS
Broadlawns Medical Center
1801 Hickman Road
Des Moines, IA 50314, USA
E-mail address: vmandracchia@broadlawns.org

ELSEVIER
SAUNDERS

Clin Podiatr Med Surg
23 (2006) xv–xvi

CLINICS IN
PODIATRIC
MEDICINE AND
SURGERY

Preface

Pediatric Foot and Ankle Disorders

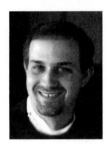

Jonathan M. Labovitz, DPM
Guest Editor

As podiatric physicians, we have the luxury of treating all systems of the complex human body and all types of patients; however, most foot and ankle conditions seen by most practitioners pertain to adults. This issue of the *Clinics in Podiatric Medicine and Surgery* is dedicated to a different patient population — that of the pediatric patient. Children are often misunderstood and may not want to talk to the doctor. They may be afraid or intimidated or they may be playing a game without explaining the rules. Often, we forget what it is like to be a child as we run behind in the office and get caught up in the self-fulfilling importance of our "adult world." In our attempt to tackle potentially complicated deformities on such a small foot, we may often find ourselves afraid or intimidated because treating the newborn, toddler, child, or even adolescent can be a relatively new task to conquer.

Then we deal with the parents. As the father of two remarkable children, Rachel and Jared, I can personally speak of the challenges of raising young children (the never-ending question Why?, the negotiations, the "art" of testing your patience, and the dreaded bedtime come to mind). But all the while, our children are our souls; what wouldn't parents do for their child? As doctors, we need to realize that the role of the parent is not exclusively that of a decision maker. There is a valuable psychologic role we play when treating the child and the parent.

This issue of the *Clinics in Podiatric Medicine and Surgery* deals with the complexity of children, whether dealing with the approach to the patient or to the examination itself. The deformities encountered can be the same as in the adult, but the complexity can be overwhelming. The dilemmas in this issue are tackled to offer new approaches to old problems. Nationally and internationally respected authors of all backgrounds have contributed in their specific areas of expertise. Some authors offer us a simplified approach and treatment, whereas others offer insight into new and potentially controversial techniques. This issue also looks into the minds of some of the field's most experienced surgeons through a round table discussion of a variety of pediatric cases.

I would like to thank each of the authors who contributed to this text. Their dedication to teaching and furthering our abilities takes a strong desire and countless hours. Each of the authors contributed to my development and I trust they will offer each of you some insight into the pediatric patient. To my wife and children, I thank you for allowing me to spend the countless hours away from you while compiling this project.

Jonathan M. Labovitz, DPM
3400 Lomita Blvd., #403
Torrance, CA 90505, USA
E-mail address: dr_labovitz@feetandankles.com

ELSEVIER
SAUNDERS

Clin Podiatr Med Surg
23 (2006) 1–22

CLINICS IN
PODIATRIC
MEDICINE AND
SURGERY

History and Lower Extremity Physical Examination of the Pediatric Patient

Jeffrey Y. Yung, DPM[a,b,c,*], Jarrod M. Shapiro, DPM[d]

[a]Residency Training Committee, Botsford General Hospital, 21111 Middlebelt Road,
Farmington Hills, MI 48336, USA
[b]Michigan State University
[c]Baja Project for Crippled Children
[d]Department of Podiatry, Botsford General Hospital, 28100 Grand River Avenue, Suite 200,
Farmington Hills, MI 48336, USA

Since Hippocrates casted his first clubfoot patient, medical practitioners of all specialties have been aware of the unique demands of the pediatric patient. As modern medicine advances, new pediatric examination techniques are added and established methods are proved, yet each technique has its own methods and pitfalls. To prevent these hazards, standardized methods of history taking and examination exist that when mastered, are comfortable, efficient, and yield successful clinical results. The purpose of this discussion is to provide a framework with which to accurately examine the pediatric patient who has foot and ankle disorders.

History

Eliciting a complete history is considered the most important component in the diagnosis of pediatric disease [1]. An accurate history affords the physician an opportunity to make a presumptive diagnosis in most cases. The pediatric history differs from the adult version, in that a birth history is included. Birth history may be divided into three distinct time periods: pregnancy, perinatal, and neonatal. Salient points to elicit include any vaginal bleeding or threatened abortion. Were any infections treated during pregnancy? Was the mother exposed to radiation or ingested toxins? Was trauma involved, especially striking the abdominal wall or

* Corresponding author. Residency Training Committee, Botsford General Hospital, 21111 Middlebelt Road, Farmington Hills, MI 48336.
E-mail address: surfmonk12@medscape.com (J.Y. Yung).

0891-8422/06/$ – see front matter © 2006 Elsevier Inc. All rights reserved.
doi:10.1016/j.cpm.2005.10.006   *podiatric.theclinics.com*

significant blood loss? Was an absence of fetal movement diagnosed during pregnancy, which may indicate arthrogryposis multiplex or Werdnig-Hoffmann disease [2]?

During the perinatal period, length of pregnancy/prematurity, duration of labor, and birth weight and length should be elicited. Was a breach birth or fetal distress experienced? Breach birth increases the risk of congenital hip dysplasia [2]. Was the labor spontaneous or induced and why? Was the delivery standard or by way of cesarean section?

An Apgar score at 1 minute and recovery scores at 5 and 10 minutes is often helpful to gather a picture of the newborn's general neonatal health. Most parents, however, are unlikely to know these values. Were any neonatal complications such as jaundice or the need for oxygen encountered? Hypoxic situations should raise the red flag of cerebral palsy.

Other important questions include history of asthma, prior dermatologic lesions, persistent growing pains, abnormal shoe wear patterns, and sleeping and sitting positions. Certain positions, such as the "W," or reverse Tailor's position, may place the child at increased risk for metatarsus adductus deformity [3], tibial torsion, or other positional or structural abnormalities.

Information regarding drug and food allergies, surgical history, and family history may also be significant. Is a family history of orthopedic or neurologic disease present? Do any family members have a history of flatfoot or cavus foot deformity? In a patient who has an erythematous plaquelike lesion, the diagnosis of atopic dermatitis is greatly strengthened by a family history of asthma or allergic rhinitis [4].

A thorough social history and medication list also assists the practitioner with attaining a diagnosis in many instances. Receipt of recent prescription medications, for example, may increase one's index of suspicion for drug reactions. In addition, recreational drug use, pets, changes in activity, changes in shoe gear, recent insect bites, and travel history may prove important in many instances.

Finally, knowledge of developmental milestones including gross motor (Table 1), fine motor, social, and cognitive skills is of considerable importance.

To further assist with ascertaining history and to facilitate the physical examination the following tactics can be employed: place the child in the parent's

Table 1
Physical milestones and associated time periods

Milestone	Age of acquisition
Lifts head	6 wk
Reaches	3–4 mo
Rolls over	4–6 mo
Crawls	5–6 mo
Grasps	7 mo
Sits	7 mo
Pulls up	10 mo
Walks	12–15 mo
Runs	24 mo

lap, maintain eye contact during the examination, avoid wearing the white lab coat, distract the child with objects, and allow them to play with examination tools (hammers, keys, etc).

Physical examination

The physical examination ideally follows a well-organized format that is performed systematically each time, preventing omission of important physical findings. Included in Fig. 1 is a history and physical template used at the Baja Project for Crippled Children. Readers are encouraged to create a similar template to permit a thorough pediatric evaluation.

A

Baja Project for Crippled Children
Pediatric Lower Extremity
History and Physical

Name: _____ *Age:* _____ *Date:* _____

Chief Complaint: _____

History

HPI: _____
_____
_____
_____

Birth History
Antenatal (Infection, bleedings during pregnancy, drainage): _____
_____

Perinatal (C-section, anoxis, trauma, breech, trauma): _____
_____

Postnatal (Respiratory problems, hospital stay): _____
_____

Birth weight: _____

Post Medical History:
Illnesses: _____
Medications: _____
Allergies: _____
Surgeries/Operations: _____
_____

Milestones of Development:
Head raise (6 wks): _____   Crawl (5-6 mos): _____
Sitting (7 mos): _____   Walking (12-15 mos): _____
Talking (18-24 mos): _____   Running (24 mos): _____

Fig. 1. (*A–C*) Standard pediatric history and physical form used at the Baja Project for Crippled Children. (Courtesy of the Baja Project for Crippled Children, Mexicali, Mexico.)

B
Physical Exam :

A. *Vascular:*

	Left	Right
Pulses: Dorsalis pedis	_____	_____
Posterior rib :	_____	_____
Capillary filling time:	_____	_____
SVPVT :	_____	_____
Pedal Hair (-/-)	_____	_____
Edema (+/-)	_____	_____

B. *Dermatological:* _____

_____

C. *Neurological:*

Primitive reflexes present –

Placement (birth-4 wks) : _____	*Moro (birth-3mos) :* _____	
Asymmetric flex/extend (birth – 4 wks) : _____		
Suckling (birth- 4mos) : ____	*Parachute sign (birth–7 mos) :* ____	
Palmar reflex (birth- 4mos) : ____	*Plantar reflex (birth-9mos) :* ____	
Babinski (absent after 2 yrs) : ____	*Assym. tonic neck reflex (6mos) :* ____	

Light touch (ant. spinothalamic tract) : _____
Sharp/dull (lat. spinothalamic tract) : _____
Proprioception (posterior column) : _____
Deep tendon reflexes (posterior root ganglion) :

           Achilles (1-4):   L- _____   R- _____
           Patellar (1-4):   L- _____   R- _____
    Clonus (sustaining or diminishing) : _____   Rigidity (fatigable?) : _____

D. *Musculoskeletal:*

Hip Examination :
Faber (present of absent of flexion, abduction, external rotation) : _____
    Ortallani's Sign : _____   Barlow's sign : _____
    Anchor sign : _____   Galeazzi's sign : _____   Telescoping : _____

Muscle strength (1-5) :

		Left	Right
Thigh :	Adductors (medial thigh) :	_____	_____
	Adductors (gluteals) :	_____	_____
	Flexors (Psoas maj. iliscus, sartotius)	_____	_____
	Extensor (quads):	_____	_____
	Flexors (hamstrings):	_____	_____
Anterior leg:	Tibialis anterior:	_____	_____
	Ext. Dig. Longus:	_____	_____
	Ext. Hallucis Longus:	_____	_____
	Per. Tertius:	_____	_____
Posterior leg:	Tibialis posterior:	_____	_____
	Flex. Dig. Longus:	_____	_____
	Flex. Hal. Longus:	_____	_____
	Gastroc:	_____	_____
	Soleus:	_____	_____
Lateral leg:	Per. Longus:	_____	_____
	Per. Brevis:	_____	_____
Intrinsics:	Ext. Dig. Brevis:	_____	_____
	Abd. Dig. Quinti:	_____	_____
	Flex. Dig. Brevis:	_____	_____
	Limb Girth :	_____	_____
	Limb Length :	_____	_____
	Length above patella:	_____	_____
	Length below patella:	_____	_____

Fig. 1 (*continued*).

Vascular

The vascular examination in children is oriented less toward searching for peripheral arterial disease and more toward screening for vascular masses, malformations, and edema. Checking for pulses, however, remains an important

C

E. Biomechanical:

Range of Motion :

		Left	Right
Hip:	Internal (extended):	_____	_____
	External (extended):	_____	_____
	Internal (flexed):	_____	_____
	External (flexed):	_____	_____
Knee position:			
	Valgum/Varum (?):	_____	_____
	External/Internal (?):	_____	_____
	Sagittal plane (genu recurvatum?):	_____	_____
Thigh-foot cods (ribial torsion):		_____	_____
Malleolar position:		_____	_____
Ankle:	Dorsiflexion (knee extended)	_____	_____
	Dorsiflexion (knee flexed):	_____	_____
Subtalar joint:	Inversion:	_____	_____
	Eversion:	_____	_____
	Total ROM:	_____	_____
	High / low axis?:	_____	_____
Midtarsal joint:	Adducted/abducted?:	_____	_____
	FF to RF:	_____	_____
First ray position:	Dorsiflexed:	_____	_____
	Plantarflexed:	_____	_____
	Hypermobile?:	_____	_____
First MPJ:	Dorsiflexed:	_____	_____
	Plantarflexed:	_____	_____
	Total ROM:	_____	_____

Gait examination : _____

_____

F. Radiological Findings: _____

_____

G. Other Physical Findings (HEENT, abdomen, genitalia, etc.): _____

_____

Impression (TEV-intrinsic/extrinsic, vertical talus, calcaneovalgus, spastic/rigid eqinus, etc):

Plan/Treatment (Casting, surgery, shoes/bracing, etc.):

Fig. 1 (*continued*).

finding to document. Temperature and color changes may be present in Raynaud's syndrome (when a primary disease is absent) or phenomenon, often identified in patients who have rheumatic diseases such as rheumatoid arthritis and systemic lupus erythematosus.

Dermatologic

The dermatologic examination of the infant varies somewhat from the older child and adolescent. Infants should be checked for dermal stigmata of spinal

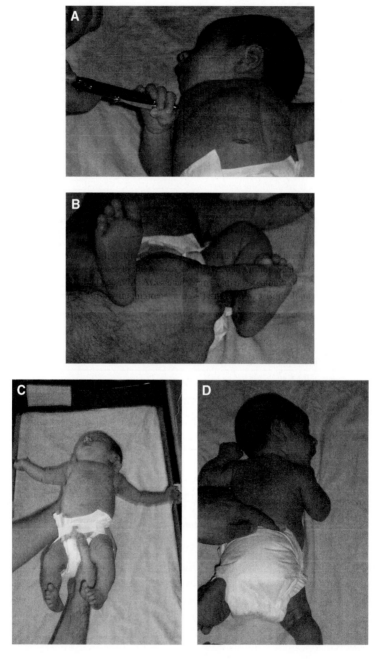

Fig. 2. Normal examination techniques and findings of common primitive reflexes. (*A*) Palmar grasp. (*B*) Plantar grasp. (*C*) Moro. (*D*) Gallant. (*E*) Vertical suspension. (*F*) Rooting. (*G*) Sucking. (*H*) Asymmetric tonic neck. (*I*) Crossed extension.

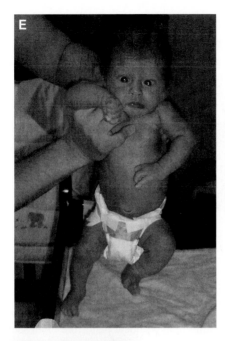

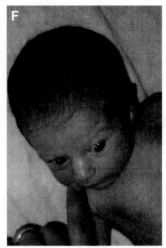

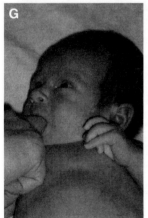

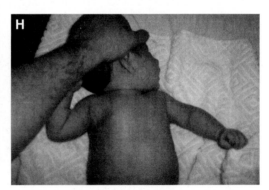

Fig. 2 (*continued*).

dysraphisms such as spina bifida. Signs of spinal dysraphisms include hypertrichosis, a hair tuft above the gluteal fold, a midline lipoma or hemangioma, or a large midline dimple above the gluteal crease [2]. A simian crease and an increased first web space with a longitudinal furrow on the foot may be seen on the palms and soles, respectively, of patients who have Down syndrome [5].

Children are often seen for podiatric treatment of dermatoses such as psoriasis and dermatitis. It is important to inspect the entire body for other signs of der-

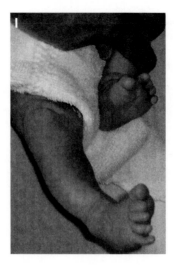

Fig. 2 (*continued*).

matologic disease. For example, psoriatic lesions may be present on extensor surfaces of the legs and arms [4]. In addition, hyperlinear palms are often seen in children who have atopic dermatitis and concomitant icthyosis vulgaris [6,7].

Congenital talipes calcaneovalgus or equinovarus show redundant skin folds and fissures in specific areas depending on the type and severity of contractures.

Neurologic

Neurologic examination of the older child and adolescent is comparable to the adult version. As such, the focus of this section is on examination of newborns to toddlers. An important concept to consider is the cephalic to caudal ("head to tail") direction of neural development, paralleling neural myelination. Therefore, developmental milestones including reflexes mirror maturation of the nervous system [4].

Primitive reflexes are brainstem mediated [8] and must be lost prior to normal voluntary control for normal development to occur (Fig. 2). Table 2 lists the most commonly tested infantile reflexes, Fig. 2 demonstrates these associated reflexes. Most of these primitive reflexes disappear by the first 6 months of life [9].

In addition, extensor responses are evoked. In the adult, this response is typically elicited through Babinski's reflex. When positive, this test demonstrates corticospinal tract disease [8]; however, some authorities argue that Babinski's reflex is more representative of pyramidal tract dysfunction [8]. This test is performed by stroking the plantar-lateral surface of the foot with a noxious stimulus and redirecting medially along the metatarsal head area. In a positive response, the toes fan out and the hallux dorsiflexes (Fig. 3).

Other extensor responses include Chaddock's (stroking the dorsolateral foot below the lateral malleolus), Schäffer's (squeezing the Achilles tendon), Gordon's

Table 2
Common primitive reflexes

Reflex	Method to elicit	Positive finding	Age range	Associated figure
Palmar grasp	Place object in infant's palm	Infant will automatically grasp object	Birth to 6 mo	2A
Plantar grasp	Touch object to plantar aspect of toes	All toes will curl downward	Birth to 15 mo	2B
Moro	While supporting the head and neck, rapidly decelerate the child by simulating a falling maneuver	Upper extremity extension and abduction followed by anterior flexion (arms fly out with hands open)	Birth to 6 mo	2C
Gallant	Scratch skin of infant's back from shoulder downward	Incurvation of trunk with the concavity on the stimulated side	Birth to 4 mo	2D
Vertical Suspension/ Standing	Hold infant upright with feet just touching surface	Infant will simulate walking motions	Birth to 4 wk	2E
Rooting	Lightly scratch corner of mouth	Lowering of the lip on the same side and movement of the tongue toward the stimulus	Birth to 3–4 mo	2F
Sucking	Place a gloved finger in the infant's mouth	Infant will vigorously suck		2G
Asymmetric tonic neck (fencer's position)	Rotate head to one side for 15 s	Extension of the arm on the side the head is turned toward and flexion on the contralateral side	Birth to 4 mo	2H
Crossed extension	Passively completely flex one lower extremity	Extension of the contralateral limb with adduction and internal rotation	Birth to 4 wk	2I

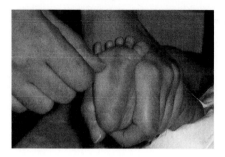

Fig. 3. Positive Babinski's reflex in the infant with fanning of the toes and hallux dorsiflexion.

(squeezing the calf), and the Oppenheim (stroking the tibia) reflexes. A positive response for all of these reflexes is identical to Babinski's reflex and is normal until about age 2 years [10].

Testing deep tendon reflexes differentiates peripheral from central causes of neurologic defects. Deep tendon reflexes are graded on a 0 to +5 scale (0 = absent reflex; +1 = trace reflex or seen only with reinforcement; +2 = normal reflex; +3 = brisk reflex; +4 = nonsustained clonus; +5 = sustained clonus).

Scores of +1 to +3 are normal, with the caveat that the findings are symmetric and no other associated abnormalities are noted. Scores of +4 and +5 are always abnormal, demonstrating clonus (a repetitive vibratory contraction of the muscle tested), a sign of upper motor neuron disease. The most commonly tested reflexes are shown in Table 3.

If the examiner has difficulty eliciting reflexes in an older child, performing Jendrassik's maneuver may be of some assistance. In this maneuver, the patient clasps their own hands, pulling them apart concurrent with the reflex hammer striking the tested tendon. Redirecting the patient's attention away from the tested area elicits a stronger reflex and more accurately categorizes significant disease.

Clonus is tested by forcibly dorsiflexing the foot at the ankle and observing for rebounding of the foot. As with deep tendon reflexes, clonus tests for upper motor neuron disease, documented by the number of repetitions or beats.

Sensory testing for the infant is limited and consists of tickling or pinching the feet. A normal infant withdraws or cries. In an older cooperative child, the sensory examination mimics that of the adult, with attention paid to vibratory, light

Table 3
Commonly tested reflexes with associated peripheral nerve and nerve roots

Reflex	Peripheral nerve	Nerve root
Achilles	Tibial nerve	S1, S2
Patellar	Femoral nerve	L3, L4
Brachioradialis	Musculocutaneous nerve	C5, C6
Triceps	Radial nerve	C7, C8

touch, proprioception, sharp/dull, and temperature sensations. In cases of unilateral sensory diminution, a dermatomal versus peripheral nerve distribution aids in determining the etiology.

Cerebellar testing is generally not performed in infants. In older children, cerebellar testing consists of Romberg's test, with the eyes open and closed. The patient is asked to stand with the feet together, with the head straight, and looking forward with arms abducted 90° to the body. The patient first keeps his or her eyes open while the clinician scrutinizes for swaying or falling to either direction, representing a positive response. The patient then closes his or her eyes, and the clinician watches for the same response. Patients who have lower motor neuron lesions, such as peripheral neuropathy, have a positive Romberg's test with the eyes closed due to loss of proprioception from damaged peripheral nerves. Patients who have cerebellar disease have a positive Romberg's test with the eyes open because the damaged cerebellum does not correctly process visual stimuli.

In addition, cerebellar testing includes finger-to-nose pointing, heel-to-shin, tandem (heel to toe) walking, and the presence of an intention tremor (tremor present only when reaching for an object).

Musculoskeletal

The musculoskeletal examination commences with inspection of the patient's gross appearance, including bulk, symmetry, and any gross deformities, proceeding through an organized and sequential format. Abnormal bulk may be seen, for example, as calf pseudohypertrophy, a common late finding in Duchenne's muscular dystrophy. Conversely, atrophy of the peroneals, referred to as inverted champagne bottle legs, is associated with Charcot-Marie-Tooth disease. In addition, overall foot appearance (cavus, planus, rectus) assists a differential diagnosis in many cases. For example, a flexible pes planovalgus foot type in a 10-year-old may be significant for a hypermobility or ligamentous laxity syndrome [11].

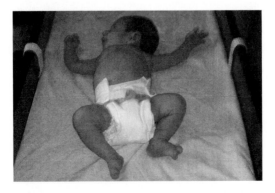

Fig. 4. Physiologic flexion of the newborn infant.

Muscle tone is defined as resistance to passive motion [12] and tested by passively flexing and extending joints of the upper and lower extremities. Normal tone is evidenced by mild resistance on range of motion. At birth, infants' natural position is one of "physiologic flexion," manifested by flexion of the elbows, shoulders, hips, knees, and to a lesser extent, the feet. In addition, the hands are in a "fisted" position. In certain disorders, such as spinal muscular atrophy, the

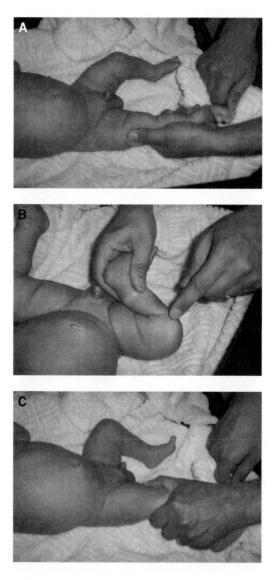

Fig. 5. Clock method of external hip rotation with the hip extended (*A*), flexed (*B*), and internal hip rotation with the hip extended (*C*) and flexed (*D*).

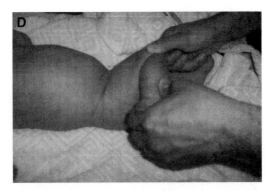

Fig. 5 (*continued*).

infant may loose the normal flexed position and appear loose, floppy, and hypotonic [6]. Fig. 4 demonstrates the normal newborn flexed elbow, hip, knee, and ankle positions and the fisted position of the hands and flexion of the digits at the metatarsophalangeal joints.

Overall muscle tone in the infant may be quickly probed with the neck flexors. Some arm resistance should be present when pulling the infant up from a supine position. At 6 weeks, the infant can hold up his or her head due to increased neck flexor strength; before this period, it is normal to observe hypotonic neck flexors. Upper motor neuron disease is evidenced by fisted hands in the older child due to extensor muscles that have not yet developed; this may be due to injury to the contralateral side of the brain. Abnormal tone is described as hypotonia (lack of tone) or hypertonia (excessive tone). Hypertonia with rigidity is best found with hip rotation and most commonly seen in parkinsonism. Hypertonia with spasticity represents an upper motor neuron lesion of the pyramidal tract and is often seen with spastic cerebral palsy, stroke, or spinal cord injury. Hypertonia with paratonia, a sign of diffuse cerebral dysfunction, is displayed by increased tone with increased force of the examiner. Hypotonia, or a lack of muscle tone, presents in lower motor neuron lesions and muscular disease [12].

Muscle strength is tested in the standard manner in the cooperative child and adolescent. Strength of the entire lower extremity should be evaluated, including all groups of the hip, thigh, leg, and foot. Muscle strength testing is documented by the Oxford scale (0 = no contraction; 1 = slight contraction, no movement; 2 = full range of motion, without gravity; 3 = full range of motion, with gravity; 4 = full range of motion, some resistance; 5 = full range of motion, full resistance) [12].

The hip examination is of paramount importance in the infant age group. Testing begins with internal and external range of motion with the hip flexed and extended. Range of motion is best examined using the clock method as described by Valmassy [13]. When visualizing the part being rotated on the face of a clock, every "hour" on the clock represents 30° of motion (Fig. 5).

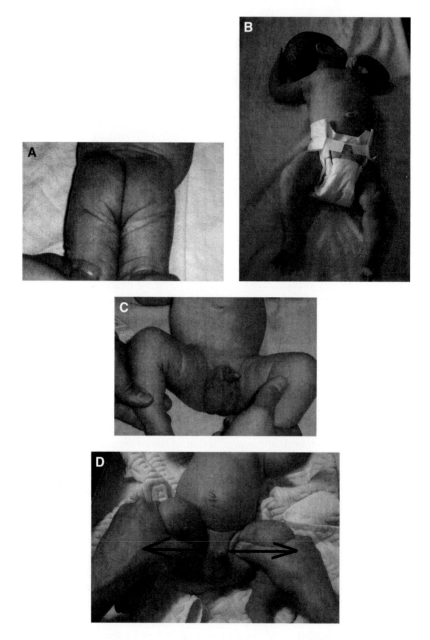

Fig. 6. (*A*) Anchor sign. (*B*) Resting hip position. (*C*) Hip abduction test. (*D*) Barlow maneuver. Arrows indicate direction of force placed by examiner on greater trochanter of femur. (*E*) Ortolani maneuver. Right hip is stabilized while left hip is abducted (attempting to reduce a dislocated hip). (*F*) Test for Galeazzi sign. (*G*) Telescoping test. Arrow demonstrates axial force examiner places on flexed hip.

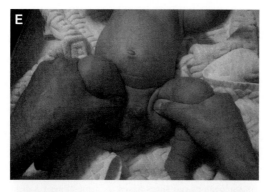

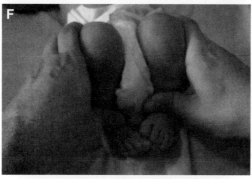

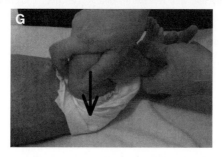

Fig. 6 (*continued*).

The clinician then proceeds to the examination for congenital hip dysplasia (Fig. 6). Tests considered most reliable include the Ortolani maneuver, hip abduction, and the Galeazzi sign [14]. Table 4 describes the various techniques for examining the infant hip. Other physical signs for congenital hip dislocation include an absence of the femoral head at the inguinal region and a normally palpable femoral head anteriorly beneath the femoral artery at the middle of Poupart's (inguinal) ligament [2]. With complete hip dislocation, the femoral head lies anterior to Nélaton's line (line drawn from anterior superior iliac spine to the ischial tuberosity) [2]. During stance, a positive Trendelenberg's sign may

Table 4
Examination techniques for intantile congenital hip dislocation

Maneuver	Method	Positive findings	Associated figure
Anchor (thigh folds)	Visually inspect anterior and posterior thigh and gluteal folds for symmetry	Extra thigh folds and an elevated gluteal fold on ipsilateral dislocated side	6A
Resting hip position	Normal hip position is flexed, abducted, and externally rotated	Affected side less rotated than nonaffected side	6B
Hip abduction	Simultaneously abduct hips, looking for symmetry	Decreased hip abduction on affected side	6C
Barlow	Tests for "dislocateable hip": Patient supine, hips and knees flexed to 90°; index finger over greater trochanter of femur, thumb over lesser trochanter; bring hips into midabduction while applying posterior and outward pressure with thumb; most reliable from birth to 4 wk	Palpable click or pop; femoral head is dislocating posteriorly over posterior lip of acetabulum; returns back to acetabulum as pressure released	6D
Ortolani	Represents dislocated (or reducible) hip: patient supine, same hand position as Barlow; hips and knees flexed; distract and abduct one hip at a time while stabilizing contralateral hip	Palpable click as hip is reduced out of dislocated position	6E
Galeazzi/Allis	Infant supine with hips flexed and knees together with feet flat on table, comparing level of knees	Dislocated side lower; more effective after 18 mo and only in unilateral disease	6F
Telescoping	Infant supine with hip flexed, adducted, and knee straight; extremity is pushed axially	Abnormal mobility or telescoping motion as femur moves posteriorly	6G

be noted on the dislocated side. When standing on one foot on the dislocated side, the contralateral pelvis drops secondary to weak hip abductors [14]. With bilateral dislocation, the perineum appears widened, and the greater trochanters are prominent [2]. Patients may demonstrate hyperlordosis, and a ducklike waddle or "sailors gait" may be present in bilateral hip dislocation, again due to weak hip abductors [2].

After examining hip range of motion and potential dislocation, the knee examination is performed. Knee position is best seen with the patient in static stance and gait. Knee positions vary during different ages as a consequence of ontologic development (Table 5). Knee positions are described as genu varum (bowleg), genu valgum (knock knee), and genu recurvatum (a posteriorly displaced knee with a posteriorly prominent popliteal fossa). A genu recurvatum of 5° to 10° degrees is considered normal until approximately age 5 years [14].

Tibial torsion is examined clinically by measuring malleolar position. A general rule of thumb for tibial torsion is to add 5 to the measured malleolar position [3]. Malleolar position is measured with the patient supine, placing the extended

Table 5
Lower-extremity positions at various ages

Hip	Knee	Tibial varum	Tibial torsion/malleolar position			Subtalar joint ROM	Ankle dorsiflexion
			Age	TT	MP		
Antetorsion	Birth: 15°–20° varum	Birth: 5°–10°	Birth	0	0	Child	Birth: 75°
Birth: 30°–20°	2–4 yr: straight	2 yr: 2°–3°	1	6	3–4	ROM: 50°–60°	3 yr: 20°–25°
6 yr: 10°–15°	4–6 yr: 5°–15° valgum	Adult: 2°–3°	2	12	6–8	15°–20° eversion	10 yr: 15°
	6–12 yr: straight		6	22	13–18	35°–40° inversion	Adult: 10°
Anteversion	12–14: 5°–10° valgum						
Birth: 60°	14–15+: straight					Adult	
6 yr: 10°–12°						ROM: 25°–35°	
						10° eversion	
						20° inversion	

knee in the frontal plane. The ankle should be dorsiflexed to 90° and the subtalar joint in neutral. The examiner's fingers are placed anterior and posterior to the malleoli to gauge the malleolar position with respect to the leg [14]. Alternatively, this same examination may be performed with the patient in the prone position. The knee is flexed to 90° and the malleolar position is compared with that of the leg by glancing axially down the leg (Fig. 7).

Next, the ankle and foot examination is performed, including subtalar and midtarsal joint range of motion, rearfoot-to-leg relationship, and transverse and frontal plane forefoot-to-rearfoot relationships. The Silfverskiöld's syndrome test is used to differentiate causes of ankle equinus. With the knee extended and flexed, the clinician dorsiflexes the ankle with the subtalar joint in neutral position and the midtarsal joint maximally pronated. When less than 10° of ankle dorsiflexion is present, the patient has ankle equinus. When ankle dorsiflexion increases with the knee flexed, the patient has a gastrocmnemius equinus. When no increase is noted with the knee flexed, the patient has a gastrocsoleus or osseous equinus, differentiated by a soft or hard endpoint, respectively. In patients who have pes cavus, stress lateral radiographs may be necessary to diagnose pseudoequinus.

The examiner progresses distally to evaluate the forefoot relationship to the rearfoot at Lisfranc's and Chopart's joints. The three primary deformities to elicit from the examination are metatarsus adductus (adduction in the transverse plane at Lisfranc's joint), metatarsus varus (frontal plane inversion and adduction of the metatarsals at Lisfranc's joint), and skewfoot (forefoot adduction and inversion with rearfoot eversion at the midtarsal and subtalar joints). Metatarsus adductus clinical findings present as a C-shaped foot with a convex lateral border and concave medial border. This condition may be evaluated by comparing the

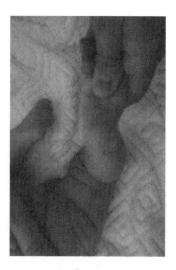

Fig. 7. Determining tibial torsion by way of malleolar position with the patient in a prone position.

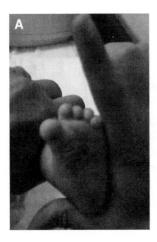
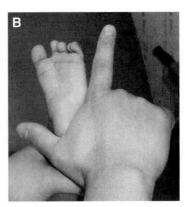

Fig. 8. Examination for metatarsus adductus. Examiner places foot into thenar space created by holding index and thumb at 90° to each other. (*A*) Rectus foot demonstrating straight lateral border of the foot. (*B*) Metatarsus adductus with curvature of lateral border in comparison with straight index finger.

lateral border of the infant's foot with the examiner's index finger and thumb held at 90° to each other (Fig. 8). When deformity is noted, the clinician should determine the flexibility by attempting to abduct the forefoot on the stabilized rearfoot.

Limb-length discrepancy should be suspected when a unilateral pes planus or hallux abductovalgus deformity is present. Although clinical measurements are highly inaccurate, full lower-extremity radiographs obtain a true diagnosis. Certain methods of examination provide the clinician with a general feel for the presence of limb-length discrepancy. Multiple examination techniques are available and include comparing the medial malleoli of contralateral limbs with the patient sitting upright against a hard surface, measuring the anterior superior iliac spine or umbilicus to medial malleolar distance, or placing blocks of different heights under the shorter side until the pelvis appears level.

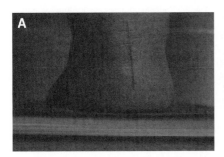
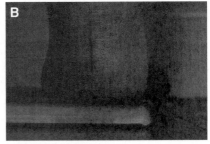

Fig. 9. (*A*) Posterior heel in RCSP. Line demonstrates varus position of heel. (*B*) Note minimal decrease in varus heel position on placement of block under lateral foot with first ray off-weighted demonstrating minimal first-ray effect on heel position in this patient.

Many experts advocate examining the patient's static stance and gait before the non–weight-bearing examination. Static stance includes determining resting calcaneal stance position (RCSP), or the position of the heel with respect to the ground. A rule of thumb for RCSP is to subtract the child's age from 7, which reveals the amount of normal calcaneal eversion [13]. For example, a 5-year-old who has an RCSP of 10° has an excess of 8° of calcaneal eversion. In addition, neutral calcaneal stance position, tibial varum or valgum, and knee position may be determined at this time. Additional static stance maneuvers include the Coleman block test for pes cavus and the Hubscher maneuver for flexibility of pes planus deformity. The Coleman block test consists of placing a block of wood approximately 0.5 inches thick under the heel with the first ray non–weight bearing (Fig. 9). If a previously inverted heel reduces to perpendicular, then heel inversion is considered secondary to a forefoot valgus deformity.

Table 6
Altered gait types and their disease associations

Gait type	Appearance	Disease associations
Steppage	Entire leg lifted at hip to assist with ground clearance	CMT, polio and postpolio syndrome, Guillain-Barre syndrome, CVA, paralytic dropfoot fascioscapulohumeral dystrophy
Dyskinetic	Uncontrolled motion while walking with athetosis, chorea, ballismus	Extrapyramidal disease
Spastic	Stiff, foot-dragging walk caused by one-sided, long-term muscle contraction	Cerebral palsy and CVA
Ataxic	Instability during single limb stance with an alternating narrow-to-wide base of gait	Due to damage of afferent nerves seen in Friedreich's ataxia, cerebellar ataxia, MS, tabes dorsalis, diabetic neuropathy, alcoholic neuropathy, and CP affecting the cerebellum
Hemiparetic	Hip circumduction and foot inversion with posturing of the upper extremity	Cerebral palsy and CVA
Trendelenberg (Waddling)	Child walks with hips, knees, and feet externally rotated	Duchenne's muscular dystrophy, spinal muscular atrophy, and dislocated hip; secondary to weak pelvic girdle muscles and hip adductors
Vaulting	Abnormally high cadence with severe lateral trunk movement and scissoring, with instability from step to step	Myotonic dystrophy
Equinus (toe walking)	Toe walking with absent heel contact	Spastic upper motor neuron diseases, benign habitual toe walking
Festinating	Slow walking with small shuffling steps with increasing cadence of steps; bent at trunk with small hurried steps; loss of reciprocal arm swing; patient has difficulty initiating gait but after starting it is difficult to stop	Parkinsonism

Abbreviations: CMT, Charcot-Marie-Tooth disease; CP, cerebral palsy; CVA, cerebrovascular accident; MS, multiple sclerosis.

The gait examination optimally occurs in an area without physical barriers and long enough to allow an unrestricted stride. As the patient walks, the examiner systematically begins at the head, observing for asymmetric tilt, then proceeds distally, inspecting shoulder height, and hip tilt. Patellar position is examined for any transverse plane malalignments. The patella should angle inward or outward, appropriate to the age group. The term *squinting patella* indicates a torsional or positional problem of the hip or femoral level [13]. If the patellar position is normal in a child being examined for in-toeing, then the rotational deformity is at the knee, tibia, or foot level [13].

The angle of gait may also provide further information. A unilateral externally rotated angle of gait may represent a congenitally dislocated hip on the same side [14]. Certain gait types are associated with specific diseases. Table 6 demonstrates common altered gait types.

Summary

The examination and treatment of children may be a highly frustrating yet highly rewarding endeavor, and the astute clinician uses all the weapons in his or her arsenal to direct a smooth process. A standardized format allows for more rapid examination and the avoidance of accidentally omitting important components that may have otherwise yielded clinical significance. An organized clinical framework to effectively examine children is the first step to successful treatment.

References

[1] Kaufman S. General examination of the infant and child. In: DeValentine S, editor. Foot and ankle disorders in children. New York: Churchill Livingstone; 1992. p. 19–35.

[2] Tachdjian M. Pediatric orthopedics. Philadelphia: WB Saunders; 1972.

[3] Volpe R. Evaluation and management of in-toe gait in the neurologically intact child. Clin Podiatr Med Surg 1997;14(1):57–85.

[4] Dockery G. Eczematous dermatitis. Cutaneous disorders of the lower extremity. Philadelphia: WB Saunders; 1997.

[5] Dubovitz V. Color atlas of neuromuscular disorders in childhood. Chicago: Year Book Medical Publishers; 1989.

[6] Uehara M, Hayashi S. Hyperlinear palms: association with ichthyosis and atopic dermatitis. Arch Dermatol 1981;117(8):490–1.

[7] Smith D. Hyperlinear palms in atopic dermatitis: a manifestation of ichthyosis vulgaris? Cutis 1984;34(1):49–51.

[8] Zafeiriou D. Primitive reflexes and postural reactions in the neurodevelopmental examination. Pediatr Neurol 2004;31(1):1–8.

[9] Grover G. Normal development and developmental assessment. In: Berkowitz C, editor. Pediatrics: a primary care approach. 2nd edition. Philadelphia: WB Saunders; 2000. p. 48–54.

[10] Harris E. Pediatric neurology. In: Thompson P, Volpe R, editors. Introduction to podopediatrics. 2nd edition. Edinburgh, Scotland: Churchill Livingston; 2001. p. 121–60.

[11] Agnew P. Evaluation of the child with ligamentous laxity. Clin Podiatr Med Surg 1997;14(1): 117–30.

[12] Kingsley R. Concise text of neuroscience. Baltimore (MD): Lippincott Williams & Wilkins; 2000.

[13] Valmassy R. Biomechanical evaluation of the child. Clin Podiatr 1984;1(3):563–79.

[14] Valmassy R. Torsional and frontal plane conditions of the lower extremity. In: Thompson P, Volpe R, editors. Introduction to podopediatrics. 2nd edition. Edinburgh, Scotland: Churchill Livingston; 2001. p. 231–55.

ELSEVIER
SAUNDERS

Clin Podiatr Med Surg
23 (2006) 23–40

CLINICS IN
PODIATRIC
MEDICINE AND
SURGERY

Metatarsus Adductus and Skewfoot Deformity

Stephen C. Wan, DPM

*Department of Podiatry, Torrance Memorial Medical Center, Suite 403,
3400 West Lomita Boulevard, Torrance, CA 90505, USA*

Metatarsus adductus, simply defined, is the abnormal medial deviation of the forefoot at Lisfranc's joint, with accompanying soft tissue contracture and sometimes resulting in adaptive remodeling of Lisfranc's and accompanying joints. Left untreated or undertreated, metatarsus adductus in the older child or young adult can progress to partially compensated or fully compensated deformities of the foot, otherwise referred to as a skewfoot deformity (Fig. 1).

Frequency and differentiation

Various authors have placed the frequency of occurrence as varying from 0.1% to 12% [1], with an even higher number for twin births and multiple births [2,3]. A somewhat weak association with concomitant hip dysplasia has also been reported [4]. However weak this association may be, a congenital hip dislocation and a hip dislocatability must be ruled out when examining a child with a metatarsus adductus deformity. Other causes of intoeing gait should also be ruled out, including hip antetorsion or anteversion, hypermobility of the knee, tibial torsional deformity, lack of external malleolar position, and talipes equinovarus (clubfoot) deformity.

Origin

Various authors have reported observations of this deformity to be accompanied by abnormal insertions of the tibialis anterior or posterior tendons, an abnormal shape of the medial cuneiform, and medial obliquity of the first

E-mail address: scwrefl@hotmail.com

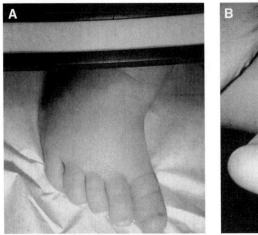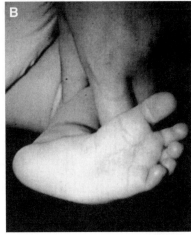

Fig. 1. (*A*) Dorsal view of metatarsus adductus. (*B*) Plantar view of metatarsal adductus.

cuneiform–first metatarsal joint [5–8]. These reports have not clearly stated whether these findings represented primary causes or adaptive changes, however.

The current dominant belief places the primary cause of this deformity as soft tissue in origin, involving muscles, tendons, and joint capsular structures, with the apex of deformity centering over the cuneiform-metatarsal articulations and with subsequent adaptive contracture leading to changes in the accompanying tendons and bones and joint structures [9].

Classification

Although flexibility is the most widely accepted criterion for classification of this deformity [10], the collective experience of the Baja Project for Crippled Children[a] has shown that the age of the patient must also be taken into consideration.

The references of clinical measurement are the "vertical" and the lateral border of the foot. The vertical is defined as the clinical bisection of the calcaneus with extension of this line distally into the forefoot region.

[a] The Baja Project for Crippled Children is a voluntary philantropic organization composed of health care professionals from the United States and Mexico who are dedicated to the care and treatment of foot, ankle, and lower leg deformities in the underprivileged and underserved infants, children and adolescents of northeastern Mexico, especially around the city of Mexicali and neighboring communities. The Baja group also strives to disseminate its collective experience and knowledge via participation in scientific conferences and the education of residents assigned from various teaching medical institutions. The Baja Project for Crippled Children has been in existence since 1973 and operates on private voluntary contributions.

The flexibility classification is subdivided into "flexible," "semiflexible or semirigid," and "rigid." It denotes that the deformity is flexible if the forefoot can be passively and easily reduced past the vertical and the lateral border of the foot demonstrates that the forefoot is abducted on the rearfoot. It is semiflexible or semirigid if the forefoot can only reduce to the vertical and the lateral border is straight. It is rigid if neither of these can be achieved.

The collective experience of the Baja Project for Crippled Children has shown that most flexible and semiflexible metatarsus adductus deformities have occurred in children 3 years of age and younger and that those children older than 4 years of age have mostly demonstrated rigid deformities. These clinical findings have also been correlated radiographically.

Radiographic evaluation

Radiographs provide valuable assessment for this deformity as a diagnostic and prognosticating tool [11]. An initial anteroposterior (AP) radiograph of the foot provides baseline values in assessment of the degree of deformity as well as in the shape of the metatarsal-cuneiform articulations. Radiographs should not be undervalued, because reliance solely on clinical assessment without the aid of radiographs may result in an incomplete evaluation. Metatarsal adduction as

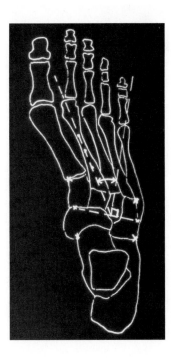

Fig. 2. Measuring metatarsus adductus using lesser tarsus bisection.

demonstrated on an AP radiograph is measured via the bisections of the lesser tarsus and the second metatarsal, respectively, or via bisection of the second metatarsal in relation to the long axis of the rearfoot (Figs. 2 and 3) [12]. Repeat radiographs after treatment (nonoperative and operative) are indicated and then at periodic intervals to monitor the maintenance of correction or any evidence of recurrence.

It is the collective experience of the Baja Project for Crippled Children that a round status of the metatarsal-cuneiform joints, as found in most pediatric metatarsus adductus deformities in children aged 3 years and younger, allows for a higher likelihood of nonoperative and operative success in correcting the deformity. In addition, the prognosis of leaving the foot relatively supple after operative correction of a "round joint" is much higher. Conversely, the success rate of a complete correction of this deformity in the "squared-off" or "adapted" metatarsal-cuneiform joints, as more commonly demonstrated in children aged 4 years and older, is lower. In addition, operative intervention in this category is more likely to create a stiff foot (Figs. 4 and 5).

The lateral radiographic view of this type of deformity typically demonstrates no abnormal findings unless (1) an improper cast immobilization technique causes subluxatory changes or (2) a rigid metatarsus adductus deformity causes secondary compensatory deformities. The latter is discussed further in the section on skewfoot.

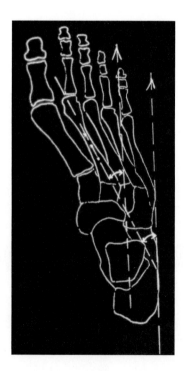

Fig. 3. Measuring metatarsus adductus using long axis of rearfoot.

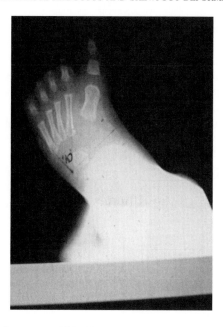

Fig. 4. AP view of a younger child with metatarsus adductus showing metatarsal bases.

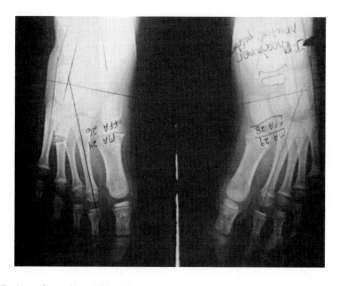

Fig. 5. AP view of an older child with metatarsus adductus showing rounded squared-off metatarsal bases.

Principles of treatment

Historically, treatment has ranged from no treatment if the deformity is flexible or unless the child develops symptoms, to waiting for development of rigidity [13], to even the outdated adage of no treatment at all, because it was believed at one time that most of these deformities would spontaneously self-correct [14]. The central theme of treatment should incorporate the following:

1. Early diagnosis
2. Early appropriate level of treatment aimed at complete reduction of the deformity
3. Prevention of recurrence.

To these ends, the flexibility of the deformity and age of the patient affect the success of nonoperative and operative treatments. The earlier that treatment can be initiated, the sooner the deformity can be resolved. Therefore, waiting and observing in the presence of a deformity, no matter how flexible it seems to be, is not advisable.

Nonoperative treatment

A flexible deformity should receive daily passive stretching from the family, typically the parents. Those rendering this type of care must be absolutely reliable and be meticulously taught the proper method of stretching. Counterpressure over the cuboid must be ensured, and the calcaneus must be left alone (Fig. 6), because unnecessary and improper pressure on the heel may lead to a valgus calcaneal position and abnormal pronation of the subtalar joint. The duration of the exercise should be a minimum of 15 to 20 continuous minutes per day over a period of at least 3 to 4 weeks and then be maintained with a pair of straight last shoes with the proper application of counterpressure padding (Fig. 7). This incorporates lateral pressure applied at the first metatarso-phalangeal (MTP) joint and medial counterpressure applied at the cuboid. Maintenance therapy should be continued for a period of at least 3 to 4 months, and the patient should be followed for at least 1 year thereafter to ensure that there is no recurrence.

A semiflexible or semirigid deformity should undergo aggressive and early use of passive stretching and serial cast immobilization. It is the experience of the Baja Project for Crippled Children that attempts at cast correction without passive stretching before each cast application significantly delay clinical results or cause rapid subluxation of the midtarsal joint. It cannot be emphasized enough to avoid valgus stress on the calcaneus. The appropriate counterpressure should be applied to the cuboid. The abductory force on the forefoot should be applied against the head and neck of the first metatarsal, the first MTP joint, and the hallux. A common error lies in not including abduction of the great toe, resulting in an occasional hallux varus as a consequence of not stretching

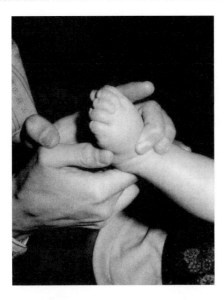

Fig. 6. Hand position in stretching the contracted structures in the metatarsus adductus. The calcaneus is not stressed. Note that the index finger of the right hand rests on the Achilles tendon and not on the calcaneus.

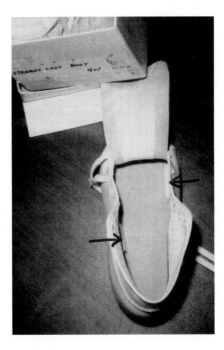

Fig. 7. Straight last shoe with padding at the first metatarso-phalangeal joint area and counterpressure at the cuboid area.

out the abductor hallucis muscle and the medial contracture of the first MTP joint capsule.

The cast should have a thin layer of cast padding, just enough to prevent pressure irritation. Too much padding is a common mistake and results in poor cast contact, thereby compromising proper correction. A slipper cast is first applied below the malleolar region, incorporating the entire foot. This section of the cast should be allowed to set while the clinician maintains the same manipulative force and hand positions as used in passive stretching. The below-knee (BK) cast segment is next applied and then extended beyond to an above-knee (AK) cast, holding the knee flexed at an angle of 45° to 60° and with the leg placed in slight external rotation. The AK cast should extend to at least midthigh or to the upper third of the thigh to avoid spontaneous "wiggling out of the cast" by the child.

A long-leg cast is recommended to avoid internal rotation of the leg on the thigh subsequent to the weight of the cast. Whether a long-leg cast shortens the length of time needed to obtain proper correction is not well established. If the child is younger than 3 months of age, weekly cast changes are advised. Biweekly changes can be used for children older than 3 months of age.

After achieving the desired correction, the child should be placed in a maintenance cast to consolidate the gains and avoid recurrence. This maintenance period should be at least one half the length of time necessary to achieve the initial desired correction. The maintenance casts should also be changed at the proper intervals. Thus, an 8-week period of casting needed to obtain the initial correction should be followed by at least 4 more weeks of maintenance casts. The final maintenance cast can be bivalved and converted to a night splint, to be worn for an average of another 2 to 3 months. Once the child can be maintained in a night splint, daytime footwear should be a straight last shoe with proper application of counterpressure padding. This is used for at least 3 to 4 months. It must be mentioned that this maintenance period represents an average. The choice to extend this period rests with the treating clinician. The child should then be followed for observation for a period of at least 1 year to ensure that the correction attained is permanent.

The use of Dennis-Browne splints or "rigid sleeper bars" as a substitute for maintenance casts is not recommended. These ready-made devices are cumbersome and objectionable from the child's and parents' standpoints; therefore, compliance would be erratic. The outdated practice of using reverse last shoes as a maintenance tool is contraindicated because these shoes abnormally pronate the foot.

The temptation to shorten the period of passive stretching, serial cast application, and maintenance casting is always present, especially when the parents start feeling the stress of the treatment process. In this author's opinion, shortening the correction and maintenance periods increases the likelihood of undercorrection and recurrence.

If recurrence is noted, timely and aggressive repetition of the previously discussed treatment processes should be instituted promptly.

The rigid deformity poses a particular challenge, because the likelihood of undercorrection and recurrence is high. Nonoperative treatment for this condition follows the pathway of the semirigid deformity, with care taken not to sublux the foot. This subluxation cause an "apparent clinical correction" when, in reality, it merely creates a secondary pathologic change to disguise the original deformity. The tracking of clinical improvement should use the combination of clinical observation and periodic radiographic evaluation. It must be emphasized that successful and complete resolution of the rigid metatarsus adductus deformity by nonoperative treatment is rare and that the likelihood of involving surgical treatment is always present. The family of the patient must thus be properly advised of this before commencement of conservative care. The Baja group, via 30 years of experience, allows 4 months as the upper limit of time to invest in nonoperative treatment for this rigid deformity. During this interval, the deformity and its possible reduction are carefully tracked clinically and radiographically. Surgical planning would commence if there is no satisfactory complete resolution of the deformity after 3 months or at the first sign of mid-tarsal joint subluxation during the same period.

Operative treatment

Although the ideal goal of treatment is to achieve full correction of the pathologic changes through the use of nonoperative treatment, surgical intervention, when indicated, should be fully entertained. It is the experience of the Baja group that spontaneous resolution rarely occurs. These claims in the past may have reflected clinical observations without taking into account the subtle but definitely present secondary changes caused by neglected or undertreated metatarsus adductus deformity. Surgical treatment should be entertained if there is no identifiable clinical and radiographic evidence of resolution after 3 to 4 months of conservative treatment or if subluxatory changes are evident on radiographs, such as forefoot abduction on the rearfoot or a breach at the medial column or lateral column of the foot.

Surgical intervention should be tailored to the specific apex of the deformity in conjunction with the age of the child.

The simplest form of residual deformity involves hallux varus resulting from tightness of the abductor hallucis muscle and/or tendon and medial contracture of the capsule of the first MTP joint. Surgical release of the tendon and capsule should adequately address this pathologic finding [15,16].

Residual medial column contracture with hallux varus can best be addressed with a combination of the previous procedure and medial column soft tissue release. The release includes a capsulotomy of the first metatarsal–cuneiform joint and the navicular-cuneiform joint, along with a release of the plantar-medial attachments of the tibialis anterior tendon [17]. Tibialis anterior tendon lengthening is rarely indicated.

Residual and resistant adduction of the forefoot for children younger than 3 years of age can best be addressed via capsulotomies of the tarsometatarsal joints and the associated intermetatarsal ligaments, as described by Heyman and colleagues [18]. One investigator has observed that between the ages of 3 and 4 years, the metatarsal bases start adapting from a round configuration to a more squared configuration. Therefore, soft tissue releases performed at Lisfranc's joint in children younger than the age of 3 years would yield a much more supple and effective correction with significantly lower rates of recurrence and incidences of degenerative osteoarthrosis. These complications are seen in this procedure when it is performed in children aged 4 years and older, because of the adaptive squaring of the metatarsal bases (H.H. Vogler, DPM, Sarasota Orthopedic Associates, personal communication, 1995).

The most common traditional method of release performed in this procedure involves a medial-to-lateral sequential approach with fixation after the releases are completed. This may result in occasional dorsal displacement of the first or second metatarsal base because of instability of the surgical sites [19]. This can be addressed by conducting the procedure in a lateral-to-medial sequential approach, however, with fixation undertaken after every two metatarsal bases have been released. Hence, the fourth and fifth metatarsal bases should first be released and fixated before proceeding on to the release and fixation of the second and third metatarsal bases, which proceeds to the release and fixation of the first metatarsal base.

In the older child (older than 4–5 years of age), this deformity can be addressed via any of the following methods:

1. Multiple metatarsal osteotomies [20]
2. Multiple metatarsal chondrotomies [21]
3. Midtarsal osteotomies with or without an accompanying release of the abductor hallucis muscle and tendon

One should be aware that an osteotomy on the first metatarsal should avoid the proximal physeal area and that an osteotomy approaching the diaphyseal region may carry an increased likelihood of delayed bony union. In addition, multiple metatarsal osteotomies or chondrotomies may disrupt the frontal and sagittal plane alignment of these structures. Frontal plane malalignment may lead to metatarsalgia of one or more metatarsals. Equally, disruption of the transverse plane parabola of the metatarsals may also lead to metatarsalgia.

In the Heyman-Herndon-Strong type of soft tissue release and metatarsal osteotomies and chondrotomies advocated by Heyman and colleagues [18], the procedures involve addressing the correction at multiple sites, with each potentially acting as a separate unit and therefore causing a higher degree of potential sequelae.

Midtarsal osteotomies, conversely, approach the correction from medially and laterally and only need to address the correction as two interrelated components. This procedure thus offers more stability and addresses the correction at the apex

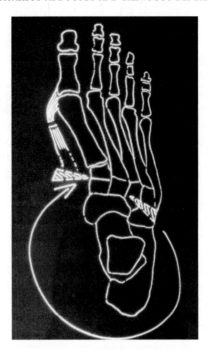

Fig. 8. Schematic diagram of the lateral closing-wedge osteotomy of the cuboid and third cunei-form, the opening-wedge osteotomy of the first and second cuneiforms, and release of the abductor hallucis muscle and tendon. Often, the wedge of bone taken from the lateral osteotomy matches the thickness of the bone wedge to be used in the medial osteotomy.

of the deformity. It has the added benefit of preserving the dominant motions of the joints of the foot, because the osteotomies only traverse the ginglymus joints of the midfoot. Some authors have advocated using separate components of this procedure independently [22]. However, the Baja group has also found that using a combination of the closing-wedge osteotomy of the cuboid and third cuneiform and the opening-wedge osteotomy of the first and second cunei-forms yields the most consistent and best long-term results in correcting this deformity (Fig. 8) [23].

Points to ponder

Certain inherent precautions should be noted in the performance of mid-tarsal osteotomies:

1. Because the cuboid is trapezoidal in cross section, a closing osteotomy through this area often results in an abduction and/or dorsiflexion of the lateral aspect of the midfoot, thereby enhancing a preexisting valgus of the lateral aspect of the forefoot. Therefore, after completion of the

initial stages of the osteotomy and before fixation, the osteotomy can be "feathered" from a plantar-lateral angle to a dorsomedial angle to adjust for a valgus attitude of the lateral column of the forefoot.

2. One must remember that the lateral component of this procedure is an osteotomy of the cuboid and third cuneiform and not just of the former, as has been occasionally and erroneously practiced. Therefore, there should be little hesitation to extend the osteotomy into the third cuneiform to achieve the proper degree of correction of this portion of the deformity.

3. Should there be a plantar osseous lip noted on the cuboid after completion of the osteotomy, this needs to be smoothed to avoid irritation to the peroneal longus tendon.

4. The medial component of this procedure involves an opening osteotomy of the first and second cuneiforms; therefore, the osteotomy should extend into the latter bone to achieve the proper corrective result.

5. Because the first cuneiform is also trapezoidal in its cross section, an opening osteotomy through this area may result in a plantarflexory position of the medial column; therefore, the bony cut can also be feathered to address this anomaly.

6. Fixation is according to the surgeon's preference and has spanned the spectrum of pins, staples, and plates.

Postoperative care

By principle, a soft tissue procedure like the Heyman-Herndon-Strong release requires an average of 6 weeks of postoperative cast immobilization. Osseous procedures, such as the multiple metatarsal osteotomies and chondrotomies and the midtarsal osteotomies, require an average of 8 weeks of immobilization. A midpoint cast change can be used for inspection of the surgical sites and suture removal. This should ideally be performed with the patient under sedation to ensure proper tissue relaxation. Pin removal for the soft tissue procedure should be no sooner than 6 weeks after surgery.

It must be kept in mind that postoperative immobilization is essentially for soft tissue and bone healing and must be followed by additional periods of cast application to maintain the surgical correction. The protocol for maintenance in terms of time, height of the cast, night splints, and shoes follows that for the maintenance of correction in nonoperative treatment.

Skewfoot deformity

This deformity is the common long-term sequela of a previously untreated or undertreated metatarsus adductus deformity with secondary compensatory changes. It is most often semirigid or rigid in the adductus component and is found in the older child, the adolescent, the young adult, and beyond. The

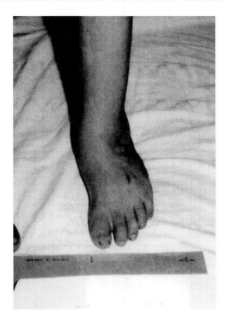

Fig. 9. Skewfoot deformity in a child. Note the adductus forefoot and the hyperpronated rearfoot.

presenting clinical signs and symptoms remarkably represent those of a pathologic flatfoot.

This deformity can thus best be viewed as a combination of a rigid adductus deformity of the forefoot region with a partially compensated or fully compensated flatfoot deformity in the midfoot and rearfoot regions (Fig. 9).

Assessment

Assessment is by clinical and radiographic means. Clinically, this type of foot most often presents with the following:

1. A juvenile bunion deformity [24] with a predominantly transverse plane subluxation of the first MTP joint [12]
2. Pain at the larger prominence at the fifth metatarsal base
3. Postural symptoms related to a flatfoot deformity
4. Occasionally, lateral foot and ankle instability

When a pathologic metatarsus adductus component is suspected in a symptomatic flatfoot deformity, the adductus deformity can be readily revealed by placing the foot in the subtalar joint neutral position (Fig. 10). Similarly, a juvenile bunion deformity should be evaluated not only by standard weight-bearing radiographs but via a weight-bearing AP radiograph taken in the sub-

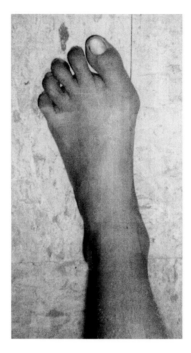

Fig. 10. Juvenile hallux valgus with metatarsus.

talar joint neutral position to assess any underlying metatarsus adductus component (Fig. 11).

As with the evaluation of primary metatarsus adductus, superstructural torsional and positional deformities in the hip, knee, and tibial regions should be ruled out.

Treatment

Nonoperative treatment is directed at the symptomatic supportive treatment of the flatfoot component. The semirigid to rigid adductus component can no longer be successfully reduced at this stage without surgical intervention. Overly aggressive manipulation or aggressive attempts at serial cast correction in an attempt to correct the rigid adductus deformity would be misguided. The use of supportive shoes and various forms of functional foot orthoses has limited application. Two investigators have postulated that a forefoot adductus angle of 17° or greater would render any form of functional foot orthoses ineffective (M.H. Root, DPM, personal communication, 1989; J.R. Weed, DPM, personal communication, 1989).

Operative intervention for the dysfunctional or symptomatic skewfoot deformity should first be directed to the correction of the adductus component

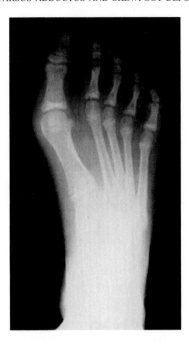

Fig. 11. AP radiograph of the same patient in a neutral stance shows adductus deformity of the foot.

and then to the correction of the flatfoot component of this combined deformity. It is this author's opinion and experience that any attempt to correct the flatfoot deformity without first addressing the metatarsus adductus component leads to protracted midfoot and rearfoot pain, gait disturbances, and other associated postural symptoms, because the body's compensatory mechanism would be eliminated by the flatfoot correction but the primary deforming adductus deformity would be left with no means of self-adjustment.

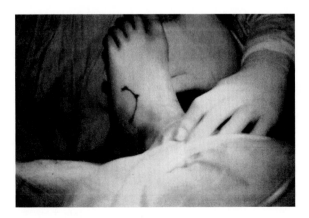

Fig. 12. One of several acceptable lateral incisional approaches to the lateral lesser tarsal osteotomy.

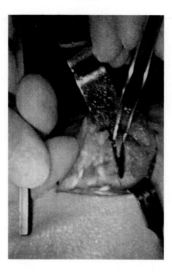

Fig. 13. Lateral bone wedge removed.

The adductus component at this stage can be most effectively corrected by midtarsal osteotomies involving the closing-wedge osteotomy of the cuboid and third cuneiform and the opening-wedge osteotomy of the first and second cuneiforms (Fig. 12). Occasionally, an appropriate release of the abductor hallucis muscle and/or tendon may be a necessary adjunct.

The surgical reconstruction of the flatfoot component, along with its evaluation and selection of procedures, is addressed in a different article in this issue. It cannot be overemphasized that the axes and planes of dominance of the associated flatfoot deformity must be accounted for meticulously. To address the flatfoot component of the skewfoot deformity via one or two preselected and routinely applied surgical procedures would be ill advised.

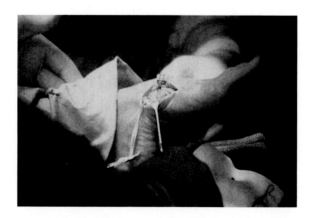

Fig. 14. Medial skin incision and exposure of first cuneiform area.

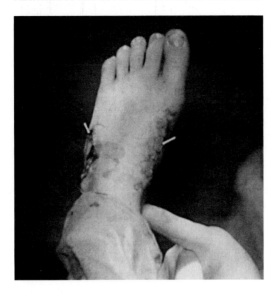

Fig. 15. Immediate postoperative clinical appearance of the foot after lateral and medial mid-tarsal osteotomies.

The postoperative care should follow the principles of bone healing as applicable (Figs. 13–15).

Summary

Metatarsus adductus deformity should be recognized and addressed appropriately and in a timely fashion so as to achieve an effective correction with low rates of recurrence. Early diagnosis and treatment are of paramount importance, because spontaneous resolution is rare. Although nonoperative treatment is desirable via manipulation and soft tissue stretching and serial cast immobilization, appropriate surgical intervention needs to be used on occasion to achieve correction of resistant cases. Depending on the severity and flexibility of the deformity and the age of the patient, various methods of surgical reconstruction are available.

A long-standing untreated or undertreated adductus deformity can lead to the formation of a skewfoot deformity with more significant symptoms and deformity. The skewfoot can best be viewed as a combination of a rigid adductus deformity of the forefoot with secondary compensatory changes in the midfoot and rearfoot, resulting in a pathologic flatfoot. Treatment of this deformity is rarely successful by nonoperative means, and appropriate surgical procedures addressing the metatarsal adductus component and the flatfoot component can be used for correction of the dysfunctional or symptomatic skewfoot.

References

[1] Wynne-Davis R. Family studies and their cause of congenital clubfoot. J Bone Joint Surg Br 1964;46:444.

[2] Hunziger UA, Largo RH, Duc G, et al. Neonatal metatarsus adductus, joint mobility, axis and rotation of the lower extremity in preterm and term children 0–5 years of age. Eur J Pediatr 1988;148:19–23.

[3] Wynne-Davis R. Etiology and interrelationship of some common skeletal deformities. J Med Genet 1982;19:321.

[4] Barlow TG. Early diagnosis and treatment of congenital dislocation of the hip. J Bone Joint Surg Br 1962;44:292.

[5] Kite JH. Congenital metatarsus varus. J Bone Joint Surg Am 1967;49:388.

[6] Browne RS, Paton DF. Anomalous insertion of the tibialis posterior tendon in congenital metatarsus varus. J Bone Joint Surg Br 1979;61:74.

[7] Morcuende JA, Ponsetti IV. Congenital metatarsus adductus in early human fetal development: a histologic study. Clin Orthop 1996;333:261.

[8] Reimann I, Werner HH. Congenital metatarsus varus: a suggestion for a possible mechanism and relation to other foot deformities. Clin Orthop 1975;110:223.

[9] Reimann I, Werner HH. The pathology of congenital metatarsus varus: a post mortem study of a newborn infant. Acta Scand Orthop 1983;54:847.

[10] Bleck EE. Metatarsus adductus: classification and relationship to outcomes of treatment. J Pediatr Orthop 1983;3:2.

[11] French S, Niespodziany J, Wysong D, et al. A radiographic study of infant metatarsus adductus treatment by serial casting. J Foot Surg 1985;24(3):222–9.

[12] Root ML, Orien WP, Weed JH. Normal and abnormal function of the foot: 355. Los Angeles, CA: Clinical Biomechanics Corporation; 1977.

[13] Rushforth GF. The natural history of hooked forefoot. J Bone Joint Surg Br 1978;60:529–30.

[14] Ponsetti IV, Becker JR. Congenital metatarsus adductus: the results of treatment. J Bone Joint Surg Am 1966;48:702.

[15] Lichtblau S. Section of the abductor hallucis tendon for correction of metatarsus varus deformity. Clin Orthop 1975;110:227.

[16] Mitchell GP. Abductor hallucis release in congenital metatarsus varus. Int Orthop 1980;3:299.

[17] Ghali NN, Abbenton MJ, Silk FF, et al. The management of metatarsus adductus et supinatus. J Bone Joint Surg Br 1984;66:376–80.

[18] Heyman CH, Herndon CH, Strong JM. Mobilization of the tarsometatarsal and intermetatarsal joints for the correction of resistant adduction of the forepart of the foot in congenital clubfoot or congenital metatarsus varus. J Bone Joint Surg Am 1958;40:299.

[19] Stark JG, Johanson JE, Winter RB, et al. The Heyman-Herndon tarsometatarsal capsulotomy for metatarsus adductus: Results in 48 feet. J Pediatr Orthop 1987;7:305–10.

[20] Yu GV, Johng B, Freireich R, et al. Surgical management of metatarsus adductus deformity. Clin Podiatr Med Surg 1987;4(1):207–32.

[21] Johnson JB. A preliminary report on chondrotomies: a new surgical approach to metatarsus adductus in children. J Am Podiatr Assoc 1978;68(12):808–13.

[22] Conklin MJ, Kling TF. Open wedge osteotomies of the first cuneiform for metatarsus adductus. Orthopaedic Transactions 1991;15:106.

[23] Anderson DA, et al. Combined lateral column shortening and medial column lengthening in the treatment of severe forefoot adductus. Orthopaedic Transactions 1991;15:768.

[24] Pontius J, Mahan KT, Carter S, et al. Characteristics of adolescent hallux abductor valgus. A retrospective review. J Am Podiatr Assoc 1994;84(5):208–18.

ELSEVIER
SAUNDERS

Clin Podiatr Med Surg
23 (2006) 41–55

CLINICS IN
PODIATRIC
MEDICINE AND
SURGERY

Talar Neck Osteotomy for Flatfoot Reconstruction: A 27-Year Follow-Up Study

Nicholas A. Grumbine, DPM

Private Practice, 555 North Tustin Avenue, Orange, CA 92867, USA

The initial study on the talar neck osteotomy was published in 1987 and contained data from 47 procedures [1]. This 27-year-old follow-up study contains the data from 215 procedures performed on 117 patients with a minimum of 1-year of follow-up. A talar neck osteotomy is performed for deformities that have an apex at the talonavicular joint or within the head of the talus [1,2]. The procedure is an osteotomy performed at the junction of the head and neck of the talus and is frequently done in conjunction with an advancement of the posterior tibial tendon and a desmoplasty to the talonavicular joint (Figs. 1–3) [1,3]. The procedure effectively corrects severe deformities that involve the talus. The correction produces a structural realignment of the talar head, making it perpendicular to the long axis of the talus. Adjunctive procedures are performed as indicated, including those cases with deformities within the posterior column [3–5] and lateral column [4,6,7]. The faulting at the navicular-cuneiform joint requires an adjunctive procedure [2,3,8,9].

Talus deformities

Severe structural deformities result when the talus is malformed and deformed or the talonavicular joint is unstable. Severe pes planovalgus and clubfeet result from malformation of the talus [1,10–14]. Instability to the talonavicular joint occurs when the talus is not superimposed on the calcaneus. The pes planovalgus

---

E-mail address: docnag@aol.com

0891-8422/06/$ – see front matter © 2006 Elsevier Inc. All rights reserved.
doi:10.1016/j.cpm.2005.10.004   *podiatric.theclinics.com*

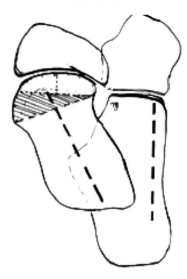

Fig. 1. The talar head-neck osteotomy site is shown on the transverse plane. The diagram shows the lack of superimposition and the deviated articular set angle of the talo-navicular joint.

deformities arising from the talus producing a talonavicular fault are medial column forefoot varus [15–17], a deviated talar head, and a long talus [1,3] producing talonavicular faulting and vertical talus and oblique talus structural malalignments [3,18–23]. Soft tissue defects affecting the talonavicular joint occur with posterior tibial dysfunction and ligamentous laxity. The clubbed-

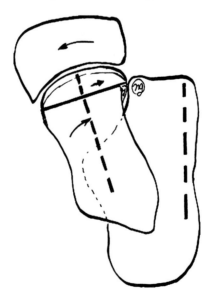

Fig. 2. The resection of the osteotomy wedge and the laterally displaced capital fragment reduces the talo-navicular deformity.

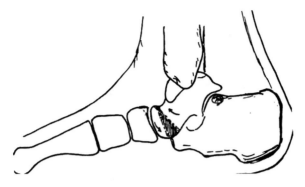

Fig. 3. The body of the talus is plantarflexed and anteriorly displaced preoperatively. The fault is at the talo-navicular joint and the head is dorsally positioned on the body of the talus.

related deformities from the talus arise from the talus failing to migrate over the calcaneus, producing a horizontal talus in the cavus and clubfeet [12,23–26].

Review of the literature

During the past 15 years, there has not been any significant new procedure developed for flatfoot corrections. The literature has presented revisions and resurrections of old procedures [1], with more clearly defined criteria for the procedures. Structural anatomy variations of the flatfoot have been described [1,11–14,27]. There have been combinations of procedures described for flatfoot deformity correction, such as the double-calcaneal osteotomy, and multiple procedures have been identified for correction of each column. The column locations of primary deformities have been identified and isolated. The posterior column pathologic changes [3–5] generate abnormal rotatory stresses, whereas those of the lateral column [4,6,7] produce stability failure. Medial column failure has an excessive adaptation that produces the arch breakdown [3,8–10].

The structural flatfoot is flat in a weight-bearing or non–weight-bearing position. A hypermobile flatfoot has a normal-appearing arch in the non–weight-bearing position and has severe collapsing of the arch with weight bearing [3,4,15,26,28]. The causes of the flatfoot are not identified by assessing the structural or hypermobile form of the foot. Abnormal medial stresses force the arch to collapse from excessive pronation. The hyperpronation produces a fault at the navicular-cuneiform or talonavicular joint [21]. The medial column breaks down, with the most severe destruction occurring when the fault is at the talo-navicular joint. The heel maximally everts, the talus diverges from the calcaneus, and the calcaneal inclination lowers. In this hyperpronated state, the midtarsal joint loses its ability to restabilize the foot. Weight bearing in this type of foot [29] maintains the foot in an adaptive state, and the arch is flattened.

The posterior column produces a flatfoot when there is spastic contracture of the triceps surae. The presence of compensating soft tissue equinus or ankle equinus produces a severe flatfoot [3,6,7,21]. A common rearfoot deformity causing talonavicular faulting is calcaneal valgus, where the heel has a lateral position and a medial center of gravity to the ankle [3–5,30,31]. When the ankle is in valgus from a proximal deformity, such as in ankle valgus, there is a talonavicular fault. The agenesis of the sustentaculum tali [32] produces medial instability from the posterior column, and talonavicular faulting results. A tarsal coalition has a diverging talocalcaneal angle that produces a rigid flatfoot with a talonavicular fault [21,29,31,33].

The lateral column produces a talonavicular fault from soft tissue when there is a spastic muscle imbalance of the peroneal brevis or dysfunction of the posterior tibial tendon [3]. The osseous deformities of the lateral column that produce a talonavicular fault occur from cuboid abduction and failure of the calcaneal-cuboid joint, with instability producing decreased calcaneal inclination, or a "rocker bottom" [3,25,30,34]. The osseous deformities of the lateral column of the compensated metatarsus adductus and metatarsus varus usually produce navicular-cuneiform faulting [3,23,27].

The medial column in a flatfoot compensates for posterior column deformities with abnormal pronation and by the breaking down of the medial arch, producing a fault. The fault occurs at the talonavicular joint, the navicular-cuneiform joint, or both joints. The breakdown of the arch results in rigid adaptive structural changes. The adaptive changes produce compression of the navicular, elevation of the medial cuneiform, and compression of the head of the talus. The talus plantarflexes [15,16,35] and the talocalcaneal angle widens with severe pronation and talar ptosis. The medial column has intrinsic structural deformities that have been well described with forefoot varus [15,16,27] and vertical talus [18,19,22,36].

Does the talus heal?

Healing of the talus has been shrouded with fear. Aseptic necrosis of the talar body is the infamous aftermath from displaced fractures of the neck of the talus [6,21]. The key is that a displaced trauma of the talar neck from the body produces the avascular necrosis. The forces required to separate the neck from the body also tear the blood supply of the talus body. The neck and head of the talus survive the trauma. Stability and anatomic reduction of the fracture are necessary to minimize the risk of avascular necrosis of the body.

The head of the talus does heal. A traumatic fracture in the head-neck region has a low risk of avascular necrosis. An osteotomy of the talus head and/or neck has an even lower incidence of abnormal healing [37–39]. The arterial blood supply to the talus head-neck region is similar to that of the first metatarsal head. The head of the talus has a rich capsular blood supply, and avascular necrosis is rare [14,38]. The wide cartilage surface on the talus head receives its nutrition through the synovial fluids. An anastomosis network from the sinus tarsi, tarsal canal, capsule, and ligaments provides the arterial supply to the talar body [40,41].

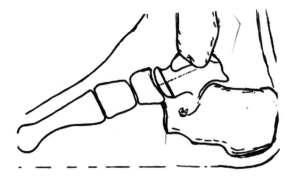

Fig. 4. After the osteotomy, the calcaneal inclination increases as the talar body dorsiflexes. The talar body becomes plantarflexed and the cyma line becomes congruous.

There are only a few reported cases of complications of surgical osteotomies or fractures in the head and/or neck of the talus in the worldwide literature [1,14,42]. The incidence of avascular necrosis of the capital fragment is rare and is no higher than the incidence in first metatarsal head necrosis. Immobilization, reduction, and adequate fixation for 6 to 8 weeks are the keys to effective healing of a talar osteotomy or fracture. The osteotomy site needs to revascularize before the stress of movement and weight bearing is tolerated (Figs. 3–6).

Talar osteotomy development

In the early literature, the major deformity of the flat foot was described as the severe collapse of the arch at the talonavicular joint. The breakdown of the arch [43] and the talonavicular faulting were treated with isolated fusions [44], fault

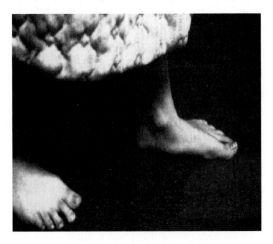

Fig. 5. The preoperative gait shows severe talar ptosis and the abductor hallucis muscle bulges medially. The fault is observed at the talo-navicular joint as the arch flattens.

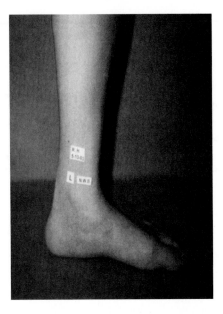

Fig. 6. 25 years after surgery, the arch is maintained at mid-stance. Adaptation is preserved at heel contact and there is active propulsion. The patient is able to stand, walk, and run.

reductions [17,45], and displacement or wedge osteotomies of the calcaneus [3,4, 19,32,34] and tendon [46,47] redirections. Soft tissues reductions for vertical talus were effective in young children [18,19,22]. In 1927, Miller [2] was the first to address the talar bulging and faulting of the talonavicular and navicular-cuneiform joints. The 10-year follow-up study by Grumbine in 1987 [1] reintroduced the talar neck osteotomy site, with 47 procedures over a 10-year period. The 1987 study redefined the deformity described by Miller [2] and tested the parameters of the procedure. The criteria were well defined for the talonavicular fault and those flatfoot deformities that occur within the talus and at the talonavicular joint [1,3,48].

Surgical morbidity reviews since the 1970s have indicated that the traditional procedures for flatfoot reduction have poor results when only the fault is reduced. Major fusions of triple arthrodesis and subtalar and talonavicular joints were the mainstay for flatfoot correction [3,21,29,33,36,43,49]. The major fusions did reduce pain and gross instability, but the trade-off was functional loss. The major fusions were an end-stage procedure.

The gross instability of the flatfoot has also been stabilized with the less destructive extra-articular arthroereisis to maintain joint function [3,21,50–52]. The goal of the arthroereisis was to reduce abnormal pronatory motion, reduce the plantarflexion of the talus, and realign the malposition of the foot without fusion. Reduction of the abnormal motion was accomplished with a bone bock or the use of an extra-articular joint implant. Enough normal motion was to be allowed to preserve shock-absorbing and adaptive functions of the subtalar joint.

Tendo-Achilles lengthening and other adjunctive procedures were used to address the primary cause of the hyperpronation. The procedure fails when the causes of the abnormal pronation are not neutralized.

Primary causes for faulting and abnormal pronation had to be reduced or controlled to achieve correction [21,29,33–36]. Calcaneal valgus [29,31], soft tissue equinus [6,7], and forefoot varus [1,15,16,27,28] were isolated components of the flatfoot complex that had to be reduced at the same time as the faults were reduced. The rare deformity of agenesis of the sustentaculum tali requires wedging of the calcaneus so that support for the talus is re-established [32]. The change of the calcaneal inclination was appreciated for the dynamics of the instability created in the flatfoot, and functional procedures were developed to change the calcaneal inclination [3,30,34].

Talus deformities

There is always a sagittal plane fault at the talonavicular joint when a talar head osteotomy is indicated. The talus is plantarflexed. The talus is also bulging medially with transverse plane instability to the talonavicular joint, and there is lack of talus superimposition over the calcaneus. Talonavicular instability is demonstrated by the navicular being poorly articulated with the talus.

Long-standing severe pronation produces structural changes within the normally rounded head of the talus. The ptosis produces abnormal compression and flattening of the lateral portion of the head of the talus as well as a deviation in the articular set angle of the talus head. The rounded head of the talus is compressed dorsally as the talus functions in a plantarflexed attitude.

The indications for a talar neck osteotomy are talonavicular faulting and a deformity within the talus. The structural deformities in the talus that produce a flatfoot are a long talus, talar ptosis, forefoot varus, and a deviated articular set angle of the talar head. A structural long talus is a congenital deformity producing a continuous medial bulging of the talar head and an anterior break in the Cyma line. A long talus requires a shortening osteotomy to the talus. Talar ptosis has a wide talocalcaneal angle and a lack of superimposition of the talus over the calcaneus. Talar ptosis is corrected with lateral transposition of the capital talus fragment. Forefoot varus from the medial column has a fixed inverted position of the medial forefoot when examined with the rearfoot in a neutral position. Forefoot varus occurs when the head of the talus fails to undergo the normal valgus rotation or there is adaptive dorsal compression of the head of the talus. Forefoot varus is reduced with a plantar wedge from the head of the talus or with valgus rotation to the capital fragment. The deviated articular set angle develops from long-standing deviation of the talus during the growing years or is congenital. The deviation of the articular set angle must be corrected to reduce the flatfoot effectively with an abductory wedge from the head of the talus. There can be multiple defects in the talus that require an osteotomy of the talus to be multiply planed.

Weight-bearing radiographs of the structural flatfoot involving the talus always have a severe talonavicular fault as seen on the lateral projection. There is a large plantarflexion of the talus, and the lateral talocalcaneal angle is abnormal. The Cyma line is broken interiorly. The calcaneal inclination angle is decreased. The dorsal-plantar view shows that with weight bearing, there is a lack of super-imposition of the talus over the calcaneus, the talus is in ptosis, and the forefoot is abducted on the rearfoot. There are significant adaptive changes from the severe pronation with the navicular-cuneiform faulting, the wedge-shaped navicular, and the angular changes within the talus.

Clinically, the arch appears low in the stance position. There is a bulging of the head of the talus medially from the talar ptosis. The forefoot is abducted on the rearfoot, and the heel is severely everted. There is a lateral bowing and positioning of the Achilles tendon. The posterior and anterior tibial tendons are distended from their retinaculum. Faulting is noted, with collapse of the medial arch.

Open kinetic chain evaluation reveals that the medial column faults are palpable at the talonavicular joint and possibly at the navicular-cuneiform joint. The subtalar joint has a tendency to evert as the forefoot is loaded. The heel has a lateral position to the malleolar bisection, and the Achilles tendon bows laterally. There is soft tissue restriction of ankle dorsiflexion when the subtalar joint is in a neutral position and the knee is extended. The forefoot is inverted to the rearfoot when the subtalar joint is in a neutral position. In the neutral calcaneal stance position, the medial forefoot is off the ground.

Abnormal compensation is obvious during gait examination. The heel strike is usually everted. The forefoot is abducted on the rearfoot, and the angle of gait is significantly abducted. The heel-off is delayed. As the medial arch collapses, faulting occurs and there is severe talar ptosis. There is no significant propulsion, because the heel remains everted at toe-off.

Biomechanical control is poor when the deformity is significant. Orthotics cause medial arch irritation as the pronation continues and the patient slides off the medial aspect of the orthotic. Shoes have a tendency for the medial counter and heel to break down and distort the shoe.

Radiologic findings of the long talus are demonstrated in the relaxed stance position with the anteriorly displaced Cyma line and the plantarflexion of the talus.

The long talus continues to demonstrate the anterior break in the Cyma line in the neutral stance position. There is a disparity between the medial and lateral column lengths. The postoperative position of a long talus reduction has the Cyma line congruous in the dorsal-plantar and lateral views.

Procedure

The talar neck osteotomy is a medial column–stabilizing procedure [1,3,48]. Exposure is made from the medial aspect of the arch and allows for exposure to the navicular-cuneiform joint, the talonavicular joint, the spring and tibial navicular band ligaments, and the posterior tibial tendon. The talar osteotomy is performed at the junction of the head and neck of the talus. The talar neck osteotomy is through and through or has a bony hinge yet maintains a hinge of capsular tissue. The wedge of bone is resected from the osteotomy site, reducing the deformity. The capital fragment is displaced to realign the head with the body of the talus. The talus is shortened as needed to create a congruous Cyma line. The osteotomy site is stabilized with two directions of fixation to prevent displacement and rotation.

The ligamentous and soft tissues of the tibial navicular band and the spring ligament and the talonavicular capsule are distended and weakened from the flatfoot deformity. The talonavicular desmoplasty portion of the procedure repairs the soft tissue as the tissues are advanced, tightened, and plicated to reinforce the medial arch. The Kidner procedure repairs the posterior tibial tendon and distally advances and tightens the tendon to the navicular and first cuneiform to create effective stabilization of the subtalar, medial midtarsal, and navicular-cuneiform joints. A Kidner-Young modification is used to repair the tendons when the anterior tibial tendon is distended from its retinaculum.

The sequence of surgical procedures follows the columns and progression of weight bearing. The posterior column is realigned first, correcting the calcaneal displacement, followed by correction of the equinus. The lateral column is then corrected as needed. Suture preference is per the surgeon's preference. Finally, the medial column is reduced. Verification of pin placement and deformity reduction is recommended through radiologic examination.

The dressings are changed in a sterile manner as soon as possible within a few days after surgery. A below-the-knee posterior splint or a bivalve cast is applied during surgery. Adequate padding is required around the external pin. The foot-to-ankle position is held slightly plantarflexed without pressure on the medial arch. Sutures are removed after 7 to 21 days as indicated by wound healing.

The immediate management of the patient requires non–weight-bearing immobilization in a cast, splint, or cast boot for 6 to 8 weeks. Gradual weight bearing starts only after bone healing has progressed for the osteotomy and any fusion. This weight-bearing transition is assisted with crutches or a walker as needed. Removal of the external pins occurs before the immobilization is discontinued. The immobilization usually lasts for approximately 9 to 12 weeks after surgery.

Early range of motion is implemented as soon as the surgical pins are removed, even though immobilization continues with a cast boot. Contrast soaking is used to reduce swelling, and the scars are softened with deep tissue mobilization. Disuse atrophy is to be expected after surgery, and strengthening exercises are implemented. Exercises for muscle re-education and gait training are necessary.

Follow-up study

A retrospective review of 215 procedures in 117 patients was conducted between 1976 and 2004. A minimum of 1 year of follow-up was necessary for in-

Table 1
Data

	No. patients	No. procedures	Follow-up (range)
Age (15 years [2–73 years])	117	215	9.4 years (1–27 years)
Sex (53 male, 62 female)		19 unilateral	
		196 bilateral	

clusion in the study. Patient age ranged from 2 to 73 years, and most patients were female (Table 1). Subjective (Table 2) and objective (Table 3) results were evaluated, revealing that 83.3% of patients achieved a good or excellent outcome.

Adjunctive procedures

With a major flatfoot deformity, multiple columns are commonly involved. Each major deformity has to be reduced in the flatfoot to stabilize and neutralize deforming forces and produce effective reduction of the flatfoot. In the medial column, additional deformities may be present in addition to the talonavicular faulting. A navicular-cuneiform fault or elevatus of the first cuneiform may be present [2,3]. The anterior tibial tendon may be distended from its retinaculum [3,48]. These significant medial column deformities need to be reduced along with the talonavicular reduction.

The medial column had significant faulting at the metatarsal-cuneiform joint or the navicular-cuneiform joint in 67.9% of the talar osteotomy procedures. The faulting was reduced with an osteotomy of the cuneiform in 5.6% of the talus procedures, and the navicular underwent an osteotomy in 25.1% of the talus procedures. A fusion was required at the navicular-cuneiform joint in 33.9% of the cases. The anterior tibial tendon was dysfunctional from distention and was repaired 95.6% of the time (Table 4).

Lateral column procedures were performed with the talar neck osteotomy in 56 feet, or 26% of the cases. A severe rocker bottom foot was addressed when

Table 2
Subjective results of the talar osteotomy

Grade	Definition	No. feet	Percentage
Excellent	No residual deformities, full ROM and activities, postural changes are reversed	58	26.9%
Good	Full ROM and activities with slight residual structural or postural changes	121	56.4%
Fair	Substantial improvement but some significant residual deformity or restriction of motion	23	10.7%
Poor	Some improvement with major restriction of motion or substantial residual deformity	10	4.6%
Failure	No improvement of function, major instability, significant pain	3	1.4%

Abbreviation: ROM, range of motion.

Table 3
Objective results

Radiograph Measurements	Calcaneal inclination angle	Preoperative	11.3 (−4–16°)
		Postoperative	18.7 (10–28°)
	Talar-calcaneal angle (DP)	Preoperative	35.3 (18–45°)
		Postoperative	22.6 (15–35°)
	Talar declination angle (Lateral)	Preoperative	42.4 (37–56°)
		Postoperative	25.7 (21–36°)
Clinical measurements	Relaxed calcaneal stance position	Preoperative	11.8 everted (8–16 everted)
		Postoperative	2.4 everted (5 everted, 2 inverted)
	Forefoot to rearfoot	Preoperative	12.7 varus (7–32 varus)
		Postoperative	1.7 varus (5 valgus, 7 varus)

Abbreviation: DP, dorsal-plantar view.

the preoperative neutral stance position failed to increase the calcaneal inclination angle to less than 12°. A cuboid-cuneiform osteotomy was used when there was significant skewing present (Table 5).

The posterior column was involved in significant deformities in 205 feet in the 215 talar osteotomies and required posterior column procedures. One hundred eighty-five of the procedures had the posterior column and medial column corrected at the same time. A medial calcaneal displacement osteotomy was required in 66.9% of the cases. An equinus correction with a tendo-Achilles lengthening was involved in 18.5% of the cases (Table 6).

Cautions

A structural flatfoot in the talus is a complex deformity. The presence of a talonavicular fault is always a complex deformity. The posterior column needs to be assessed to determine its role in the abnormal structure. If present, the navicular-cuneiform fault must be reduced as the talonavicular fault is reduced. The severe subluxation and rocker bottom position of the lateral column cannot

Table 4
Adjunctive procedures: medial column concurrent deformities

No. patients	Medial column deformity	Adjunctive procedures/recommended procedures
12	First cuneiform elevatus	Plantarflexory cuneiform osteotomy
73	N-C arthrosis/instability	Miller or Hoke N-C arthrodesis with wedging
54	N-C joint fault	Navicular osteotomy
7	First M-C instability	Lapidus or Miller arthrodesis
205	Anterior tibial tendon distention	Kidner-Young suspension/anastomosis with posterior tibial tendon

Abbreviations: M-C, metatarsal-cuneiform; N-C, navicular-cuneiform.

Table 5
Adjunctive procedures: lateral column concurrent deformities

No. patients	Lateral column deformity	Adjunctive procedures/recommended procedures
39	Metatarsus adductus or metatarsus Adductovarus	Cuboid and third cuneiform abductory osteotomy or cuboid and third cuneiform abductory and dorsiflexory osteotomy
13	Rocker bottom with abducted cuboid or with low calcaneal inclination	Opening adductory Evans osteotomy or Opening plantarflexory Evans osteotomy
2	Rocker bottom with C-C prolapse	Reverse Japas or Cole osteotomy
2	Rocker bottom with C-C instability or arthrosis	Evans C-C joint arthrodesis

Abbreviation: C-C, calcaneo-cuboid.

be reduced by itself. The presence of severe skewing needs to be reduced together with reduction of the metatarsus adductus.

Restriction of motion is present before surgery, and there is the expectation of restricted motion after surgery. The reason for the decreased range of motion needs to be determined. If there is an operative coalition, the coalition needs to be resected. If severe arthrosis is present, a major arthrodesis needs to be considered. The position and stability can be improved with the correction.

Hyperelasticity, when severe, is a consideration for arthroereisis, fusions, or bone-blocking procedures. Subtalar corrections are recommended to be deferred as a second-stage procedure. There is a normal reduction of abnormal motion after the talar osteotomy procedures, and unnecessary blocking of subtalar motion is not recommended.

The talar neck osteotomy has proven to be an effective flatfoot correction when there is a talonavicular fault. The complexity of the flatfoot becomes apparent when each of the columns is taken into consideration. The reduction of the flatfoot can have predictable results when each column is assessed fully and each segment is reduced.

The earlier talar osteotomy studies reported good results; however, the results have greatly improved using more precise criteria for the medial column, accompanied by lateral and posterior column corrections.

Table 6
Adjunctive procedures: posterior column concurrent deformities

No. patients	Posterior column deformity	Adjunctive procedures/recommended procedures
144	Calcaneal valgus	Medial displacement calcaneal osteotomy
37	Equinus, soft tissue cause	(TAL)
3	Equinus, ankle	Plantarflexory calcaneal osteotomy with TAL
1	Sustentaculum tali agenesis	Sustentaculum tali opening wedge osteotomy
4	Equinus, spastic	Murphy tendon transfer (second stage)
5	Hyperelasticity	Arthroereisis (usually a separate stage)
9	Tarsal coalition	Resection of coalition (usually a separate stage)
2	Ankle valgus	Epiphysiodesis or tibial osteotomy

Abbreviation: TAL, tendo-Achilles lengthening.

Table 7
Complications

Type	No. feet	Long-term effect
Osteomyelitis	1	Triple arthrodesis
AVN talar head	1	Talonavicular arthrodesis
Delayed union/nonunion talus	3	Bone stimulator
	1	Bone graft
Restricted tarsal ROM (after surgery)	6	Decreased function and motion
Restricted tarsal ROM (before and after surgery)	3	Triple arthrodesis
Painful T-N joints	4	Tarsal arthrodesis
Significant residual deformity	21	Additional surgical correction requiring a second stage of correction

Abbreviations: AVN, avascular necrosis; ROM, range of motion; T-N, talo-navicular.

Complications define the limits of any procedure (Table 7). Infection is a risk of any operation. When an infection occurs, surgical failure can result. Complications of the talus healing in the long-term study were reduced as patient compliance increased, fixation required a minimum of 6 weeks, the patient was non–weight bearing for a minimum of 6 weeks, and two planes of fixation were used. The preoperative restriction of motion became a significant criterion for the functional correction of the talar neck osteotomy. The presence of other structural deformities was not significant as long as each column with a deformity was also corrected.

Summary

A talar osteotomy effectively reduces talonavicular faults and deformities of the talus. The talus has been proven to heal well. The deformities that involve the talus must be corrected to reduce a flatfoot with a talonavicular fault effectively. For good results, each column must be assessed and deformities must be corrected. The posterior column has a large percentage of deformities that make up the flatfoot complex. Structurally, the equinus and calcaneal valgus need to be reduced as the talonavicular joint is reduced. The lateral column deformities of rocker bottom and skewing need to be reduced. The presence of a fault at the navicular-cuneiform joint needs to be reduced as the talonavicular fault is reduced.

The alternatives to effective column flatfoot reductive surgery are destructive and restrictive procedures of arthrodesis and arthroereisis. The fusions are indicated in failed flatfoot procedures, gross instability, and painful arthrosis. The author prefers to save joints, stabilize deformities, and preserve function rather than just to stabilize a deformity.

References

[1] Grumbine NA. Talar neck osteotomy for the treatment of severe structural flatfoot deformities. Clin Podiatr Med Surg 1987;4:119–36.

[2] Miller OJ. Plastic foot operation. J Bone Joint Surg 1927;9:84–91.

[3] Marcinko DE. Medical and surgical therapeutics of the foot and ankle. Baltimore (MD): Williams & Wilkins; Baltimore; 1992. p. 477–505.

[4] Lord PJ. Correction of extreme flatfoot, value of osteotomy of the os calcis and inward displacement of posterior fragment [Gleich operation]. JAMA 1923;81:1502–6.

[5] Silver CM, Simons SD, Spindell S, et al. Calcaneal osteotomy for valgus and varus deformities of the foot in cerebral palsy. J Bone Joint Surg Am 1967;49:232–46.

[6] Sgarlato TE, Morgan J, Shane HS, et al. Tendo-Achilles lengthening and its effect on foot disorders. J Am Podiatry Assoc 1975;65:849–71.

[7] White JW. Torsion of the Achilles tendon: its surgical significance. Arch Surg 1943;46:784–7.

[8] Hoke M. An operation for the correction of extremely relaxed flat feet. J Bone Joint Surg Br 1931;13:773–83.

[9] Jack EA. Navicular-cuneiform fusion in the treatment of flatfoot. J Bone Joint Surg Br 1953; 35:75–82.

[10] Anderson JG, Harrington R, Ching RP, et al. Alterations in talar morphology associated with adult flatfoot. J Foot Ankle Int 1997;18(11):705–9.

[11] Bleck EE. Persistent fetal medial deviation of the talus: a common cause of intoeing in children. J Bone Joint Surg 1976;58:724.

[12] Hjelmstedt A. Corrective osteotomy of the talus in congenital clubfoot. Acta Orthop Scand 1984; 45:978.

[13] Hjelmstedt A, Sahlstedt I. Talar deformity in congenital clubfeet. An anatomical and functional study with special reference to ankle joint mobility. Acta Orthop Scan 1974;45(4):628–40.

[14] Huber H, Galantay R, Dutoid M. Avascular necrosis after osteotomy of the talar neck to correct residual clubfoot deformity in children—a long term review. J Bone Joint Surg Br 2002;84(3): 426–30.

[15] Root ML, Orien WP, Weed JH. Normal and abnormal function of the foot. Los Angeles (CA): Clinical Biomechanics Corporation; 1977.

[16] Root ML, Orien WP, Weed JH, et al. Biomechanical examination of the foot. Los Angeles (CA): Clinical Biomechanical Corporation; 1971.

[17] Clark WA. A rebalancing operation for pronated feet. J Bone Joint Surg 1931;13:861.

[18] Harrold AT. The problem of congenital vertical talus. Clin Orthop 1973;97:133–43.

[19] Lloyd-Robert JC, Spence AJ. Congenital vertical talus. J Bone Joint Surg [Br] 1958;40(1): 33–41.

[20] McCarthy DJ. The developmental anatomy of pes valgo planus. Clin Podiatr Med Surg 1989; 613:491–509.

[21] McGlamry ED, Kitting RW. Equinus foot—an analysis of the etiology, pathology, and treatment techniques. J Am Podiatry Assoc 1973;63(5):165–84.

[22] Osmond-Clark H. Congenital vertical talus. J Bone Joint Surg Br 1956;38:334–41.

[23] Evans D. Relapsed clubfoot. J Bone Joint Surg Br 1961;43:722–33.

[24] Turco VJ. Clubfoot. New York: Churchill Livingstone; 1981. p. 45–70.

[25] Victoria-Diaz A, Victoria-Diaz J. Pathogenesis of idiopathic clubfoot. Clin Orthop 1984;185: 14–24.

[26] Beck EL, McGlamery ED. Modified Young tendo suspension technique for flexible flatfoot. J Am Podiatry Assoc 1973;63:582–604.

[27] Grumbine NA. The varus components of the forefoot in the flatfoot deformities. J Am Podiatry Assoc 1987;77(1):14–20.

[28] Sgarlato T. Pediatric foot surgery. Clin Podiatry 1984;1(3):709–23.

[29] Jahass MH. Disorders of the foot. Philadelphia: WB Saunders; 1982. p. 532–7, 758–61.

[30] Dwyer FC. The relationship for variations in the size and inclinations of the calcaneus to the shape of the whole foot. Ann R Coll Surg Engl 1964;34:120–37.

[31] Jacobs AM, Oloff L, Visser HJ. Calcaneal osteotomy in the management of flexible and non-flexible flatfoot deformity: a preliminary report. J Foot Surg 1981;20(2):57–66.

[32] Selakovich WG. Medial arch support by operation—sustentaculum tali procedure. Orthop Clin North Am 1973;4(1):117–44.

[33] Lanham R. Indications and complications of arthroereisis in hypermobile flatfoot. J Am Podiatry Assoc 1979;69(3):178–85.

[34] Evans D. Calcaneal valgus deformity. J Bone Joint Surg Br 1975;57(3):270–8.

[35] Bleck EE, Bergins UJ. Conservative management of pes valgus with plantarflexed talus, flexible. Clin Orthop 1977;102:85–93.

[36] Tachdjian M. The child's foot. Philadelphia: WB Saunders; 1985.

[37] Canale ST, Kelly FB. Fractures of the neck of the talus—long C term evaluation of seventy one. J Bone Joint Surg Am 1978;60(2):143–56.

[38] Kenwright J, Taylor RG. Fracture of the neck of the talus. J Bone Joint Surg Am 1958;40: 1115–20.

[39] Kelly PJ. Anatomy, physiology, and pathology of the blood supply of bones. J Bone Joint Surg Am 1968;50(4):766–83.

[40] Mulfinger GL, Trueta J. The blood supply of the talus. J Bone Joint Surg Br 1970;52:160–7.

[41] Peterson L, Goldie D, Lindell D. The arterial supply of the talus. Acta Orthop Scand 1974;45: 260–70.

[42] Monroe MT, Maoli II A. Osteotomy for malunion of a talar neck fracture: a case report. Foot Ankle Int 1999;20(3):192–5.

[43] Rose GK. Correction of pronated foot. J Bone Joint Surg Br 1958;40(4):674–83.

[44] Lowman CL. An operative method for the correction of certain forms of flatfoot. JAMA 1923; 81:1500–2.

[45] Butte FL. Navicular-cuneiform arthrodesis: and end result study. J Bone Joint Surg 1937;19(2): 496–502.

[46] Kidner FC. The prehallux in its relation to flatfoot. J Bone Joint Surg 1929;11:831–7.

[47] Young CS. Operative treatment of pes planus. Surg Gynecol Obstet 1939;68:1099–101.

[48] Walter JH, Bailey MA, Kresslen MR. Sub capital talar osteotomy to correct transverse plane structural flatfoot deformities. J Foot Ankle 1995;34(2):177–82.

[49] Lawton JH. Forefoot surgery. Complications in foot surgery. Baltimore (MD): Williams & Wilkins; 1984. p. 223–41.

[50] Sgarlato TE. Subtalar arthroereisis implant. J Foot Surg 1983;22:388.

[51] Smith SD, Millar EA. The STA operations. Chicago: Richards Manufacturing Company; 1978.

[52] Subotnick S. The subtalar joint lateral extra-articular arthroresis. J Am Podiatry Assoc 1977; 67(3):157–71.

ELSEVIER
SAUNDERS

Clin Podiatr Med Surg
23 (2006) 57–76

CLINICS IN
PODIATRIC
MEDICINE AND
SURGERY

The Algorithmic Approach to Pediatric Flexible Pes Planovalgus

Jonathan M. Labovitz, DPM[a,b,c],*

[a]West Torrance Podiatrists Group, Inc., Torrance, CA, USA
[b]West Los Angeles Veterans Affairs Medical Center, Los Angeles, CA, USA
[c]Baja Project for Crippled Children, Torrance, CA, USA

Pediatric flatfoot has long been a topic that questions what is normal and what is pathologic, when to treat and when to observe, what is the best conservative treatment, and when to intervene surgically and with what approach. Staheli [1] may have stated this best when he wrote, "Flatfoot is normal in infants, children, and some adults. The single most important principle of medical practice in making a differential diagnosis of a patient with a flatfoot is to distinguish between its physiologic and pathologic forms."

Although there are many questions surrounding this topic, the surgical approach to this complex deformity has varied in many ways. The approach has involved soft tissue correction and osseous correction. There are isolated procedures, and there are combinations of procedures. Many of the techniques used are explained anecdotally. The literature is replete with articles explaining what procedures or combination of procedures worked well, but few reasons are given for the successes and even fewer reasons for the failures. Pressman [2] wrote, "It stands to reason that for flexible flatfoot there is no one universal procedure." In this article, the author attempts to incorporate some principles of the biomechanics of surgery to guide the surgeon through the complexity of the pediatric flexible pes planovalgus.

* Suite 403, 3400 Lomita Avenue, Torrance, CA 90505.
   E-mail address: dr_labovitz@feetandankles.com

0891-8422/06/$ – see front matter © 2006 Elsevier Inc. All rights reserved.
doi:10.1016/j.cpm.2005.10.001   *podiatric.theclinics.com*

Historical approach

Pediatric pes planovalgus surgery has been considered when the patient is no longer responding to conservative treatments and experiences pain, fatigue, or an inability to participate in usual daily activities. Surgeons typically proceed through a clinical and radiographic evaluation to determine the procedure(s) of choice. Historically, this approach has led doctors to develop a plan based on the anatomic location of the flatfoot and the combination of procedures they believe has worked well in the past (Table 1). Unfortunately, prior procedures that have been successful are usually based on anecdotal combinations attempted previously or found in the literature in a small sample size and, frequently, with only short-term follow-up.

The anterior calcaneal osteotomy, or Evans procedure, has been described throughout the literature as a solitary procedure or with ancillary procedures. This procedure has withstood the test of time, with numerous studies demonstrating the effectiveness of the procedure. Mosca [3] had a successful outcome in 29 of 31 patients with nearly a 3-year follow-up. Anderson and Fowler [4] reported long-term success in 8 of 9 feet in nearly a 7-year follow-up. Phillips [5] reported similar results in 17 of 23 feet over a 7- to 20-year follow-up. Despite the long-term success, Phillips reported that the procedure failed in 6 feet (26%) secondary to regression of the talonavicular displacement or a valgus calcaneus. Cohen-Sobel and colleagues [6] reported on 8 patients who were 10 years of age or older having undergone their usual flatfoot procedures consisting of an Evans osteotomy, Young tenosuspension, and tendo-Achilles lengthening. Failure occurred in 25% of the patients.

Posterior calcaneal osteotomies were first described by Gleich in 1893. Since then, numerous methods of performing such an osteotomy have been described, ranging from medial translational osteotomies to opening and closing wedge osteotomies [7–10]. Koutsogiannis [8] noted successful correction of the rearfoot valgus position. Grumbine and coworkers [9] also reported good success in 48 patients with the "L"-shaped calcaneal osteotomy, restoring the alignment of

Table 1
Procedures from historical perspective

Medial column procedures	Extra-articular calcaneus	Anterior calcaneus	Posterior calcaneus
Kidner	Chambers	Evans	Gliech
Lowman	Baker-Hill		Dwyer
Young	Selakovich		Lord
Miller	Polyethylene peg		Koutsogiannis
Hoke	STA-Peg		L-shaped osteotomy
Talar head osteotomy	MBA		MDCO
Talonavicular arthrodesis			

Abbreviations: MBA, Maxwell-Brancheau arthroeisis; MDCO, medial displacement calcaneal osteotomy; STA, subtalar arthroreisis.

the Achilles tendon and the rearfoot to leg alignment. Other studies have also demonstrated the success of the posterior calcaneal osteotomy when treating flexible pes planovalgus.

Extra-articular subtalar joint procedures most commonly refer to the subtalar arthroereisis. Initially, the procedure was done with a bone graft and has since been performed with a silastic sphere, polyethylene plug, bioresorbable material, and various metallic constructs. Mechanically, this procedure reduces the torsional forces at the subtalar joint while limiting calcaneal eversion. This new vertically positioned calcaneus relocates and supports the talar head, preventing plantarflexion and adduction [11,12]. By limiting the calcaneal eversion, the midtarsal joint should be stable and the peroneus longus tendon has a stable cuboid for normal function. Lundeen [13] reported that the arthroereisis procedure is unable to correct a hypermobile midtarsal joint, however. The arthroereisis procedure can also accentuate tibial torsion, equinus, metatarsus adductus, medial column faults, and forefoot supination [13–15].

A number of studies, usually with short-term follow-up, have reported good to excellent results, whether as an isolated procedure or, more commonly, in combination with other procedures [11,14–16]. There are some fair results as well. Addante and colleagues [16] reported two fair results and one poor result in only 10 patients. Lundeen [13] reported fair results in 19% of his patients. The patients with the fair outcomes had metatarsus adductus (n = 4) or a midtarsal breech (n = 10).

Medial column procedures involve arthrodesis procedures and combination procedures. Although the naviculocuneiform fault is the most common location of the sagging medial column, arthrodesis of this joint fails if it is performed exclusively [11]. Butte [17] reported a failure rate of 50%, defining the limitations of the naviculocuneiform arthrodesis to be severe pronation, rearfoot arthritic changes, and talonavicular fault. Seymour [18] also reported a 50% failure rate in a long-term follow-up of 15 years in 32 feet. He attributed the failures to a return of the symptoms, because the procedure is unable to maintain the corrected position of the arch. Similar results were confirmed by Crego and Ford [19] in nine patients with only a 22% success rate.

Combination procedures, such as the Miller procedure (arthrodesis of the navicular–medial cuneiform–first metatarsal joints and advancement of the spring ligament with an osteoperiosteal flap), have success in a limited patient population with a medial column fault not located at the talonavicular joint. These successes still account for only 84% of the 38 adolescent patients reported on [20]. Chi and coworkers [21] reported a failure rate of 8% in patients undergoing an isolated lateral column lengthening and 20% in patients undergoing an isolated medial column stabilization procedure.

The historical approach usually works well if most flatfeet are of the same cause, with the same available motion at the same joints and the same compensation occurring in each patient. This arbitrary designation of the patients, without regard to the surgical biomechanics, may be the cause of the fair and poor results reported in the literature.

Biomechanical approach

The author favors an approach geared toward understanding the cause of the flexible pes planovalgus and understanding the compensatory mechanics of the foot and ankle. The biomechanical approach depends on the theory of planal dominance and the center of rotation of angulation (CORA), affording the surgeon the opportunity to achieve a functional correction of the flatfoot. Although many of the anecdotal or historical combinations may still be found to be valid, this biomechanical approach does not neglect the patients who do not fit the mold to which we arbitrarily assign them. The goal is to show an alternative method of determining the procedures that would increase the good and excellent results in our patients, thus eliminating the fair outcomes.

When looking critically at the fair to poor outcomes of the historical combinations of procedures in the literature, the author notes that specific criteria have pointed the foot and ankle surgeon to the biomechanical approach. For example, in the Evans procedure, the anterior calcaneal osteotomy addresses the transverse plane component of the flatfoot [11,22].

Some authors have proposed that lateral column lengthening is capable of correcting flexible pes planovalgus without medial column intervention. A radiographic study demonstrated an improved talonavicular coverage, reduced rearfoot valgus and forefoot abduction, and improved sagittal alignment of the medial column [23]. Roye and Raimondo [24] supported this claim by stating that the Evans procedure corrects rearfoot valgus, forefoot abduction, and midfoot pronation. Medial column contact areas decrease after an Evans procedure [25]. When evaluating the pediatric population, Anderson and Fowler [4] concluded that the Evans procedure can be done alone, because forefoot supination spontaneously corrects in the younger child. These investigators also determined that lateral column lengthening insufficiently corrects a flatfoot if done alone, however. Anderson and Fowler [4] reported the need for additional procedures in the older child. Additionally, the medial column fault and the frontal plane deformity do not resolve after an Evans procedure, especially in the older child [11,26]. This may explain the sagittal plane and frontal plane failures of Phillips [5] and the 9% failure rate of Davitt and coworkers [25] despite the normal radiographic parameters after surgery. The failures reported by Davitt and coworkers [25] were attributed to poor functional outcome.

Although some authors have determined that forefoot supinatus may be reduced with the posterior calcaneal osteotomy and that the talo–first metatarsal angle improves, suggesting correction of midfoot pathologic conditions, others have debated this theory [8,27]. Some have stated that the posterior calcaneal osteotomy frequently fails if performed alone, because the frontal plane correction does not address midfoot pronation or forefoot abduction [4,24]. Although Grumbine and coworkers [9] noted that the "L"-shaped calcaneal osteotomy corrects triplanar deformities based on proper wedging of the osteotomy, the study only evaluated rearfoot-to-leg and subtalar joint parameters clinically and radiographically. The study does note that adjunctive procedures were necessary to address midfoot and forefoot pathologic findings despite potential triplanar correction. Additionally, although the calcaneus may be in better alignment in comparison to the leg, the subtalar joint may remain maximally pronated [28]. This may account for the 25% failure rate to restore the medial column arch height reported by Koutsogiannis [8]. Catanzariti and colleagues [29] reported that seven failures (n = 24) were the result of severe preoperative radiographic findings, leading to the conclusion that posterior calcaneal osteotomies cannot adequately correct the more severe deformities.

The subtalar arthroereisis results in fair outcomes when the procedure is done in a transverse plane–dominant patient, because the arthroereisis procedure is geared toward the frontal plane deformity. In the transverse plane–dominant flatfoot patient, an arthroereisis produces a supinated and unstable rearfoot with pain [12]. Lundeen's failures occurred in transverse plane and sagittal plane deformities [13]. Finally, the medial column procedures have mixed results, and each procedure has specific limitations. These limitations have pointed to the procedure being performed away from the apex of the deformity and the failure to stabilize adequately the locking mechanism of the midtarsal complex that occurs with pronation [17,18,20,30].

Planal dominance

Planal dominance addresses each of the three cardinal planes by determining which of the plane(s) compensates for the deformity (Table 2). The primary plane of compensation and the amount of available motion are the important considerations when evaluating the dominant plane. The foot functions as a unit based on the motion and resultant planal dominance of the subtalar joint, ankle joint, and midtarsal joint [31]. An understanding of the orientation of the joint axis, and thus an understanding of the joint motion, is necessary for a true understanding of the theory of planal dominance.

Motion in a ginglymus (hinge) joint occurs at the junction of the planes perpendicular to the plane of motion. For example, if the motion is exclusively seen in the frontal plane, the motion occurs at an imaginary hinge at the junction of the transverse plane and sagittal plane. If the motion were not exclusively frontal plane motion, the hinge would not be located exactly at the junction of the transverse and sagittal planes.

Table 2
Determining planal dominance on radiographs

Sagittal plane	Frontal plane	Transverse plane
↑ Talar declination angle	↓ First metatarsal declination angle	↑ Talocalcaneal angle (AP)
↑ Talo-calcaneal angle (lateral)	↓ Height sustentaculum tali	↑ Calcaneocuboid angle
↓ Calcaneal inclination angle	↑ Superimposition lesser tarsus	↓ Talonavicular congruency
Naviculocuneiform breach	(lateral)	↓ FF to RF adduction
	Widening lesser tarsus (AP)	

Abbreviations: AP, anteroposterior; FF, forefoot; RF, rearfoot; ↑, increased; ↓, decreased.

The subtalar joint axis is located 42° to the frontal plane and transverse plane and 16° to the sagittal plane. There is virtually an even amount of frontal plane motion (inversion-eversion) and transverse plane motion (abduction-adduction) in the normal foot, meaning that for each degree of calcaneal eversion, there is 1° of talar adduction. There is more inversion-eversion and virtually no abduction-adduction if the joint axis becomes more horizontal. The lower joint axis creates frontal plane dominance at the subtalar joint. The frontal plane dominance causes an unlocking of the calcaneocuboid joint, making the midtarsal joint unstable. Secondary compensation then occurs, because the motion is in response to the excessive eversion at a triplanar joint. Dorsiflexion and eversion constitute the secondary motion at the midtarsal joint, whereas the subtalar joint has a loss of the calcaneal inclination.

A more vertically oriented subtalar joint axis, or a high joint axis, limits the frontal plane motion and creates more transverse plane motion. When this dominant transverse plane situation occurs, there can be a severely pronated foot clinically with a relatively normal calcaneal inclination. There is limited sagittal plane motion, because the joint axis is virtually parallel to the sagittal plane. The subtalar joint axis lies closer to the frontal and transverse planes when the sagittal plane is the dominant plane of compensation. The ankle joint usually generates sagittal plane motion. The ankle joint axis is oriented in the same direction as the subtalar joint, and it is 84° from the sagittal plane of the foot, making it the dominant plane at the ankle.

The midtarsal joint is composed of two individual joints, which combine to form Chopart's joint. The talonavicular joint and calcaneocuboid joint have individual functions, but they also work in concert for a combined function. Individually, the talonavicular joint belongs to the talocalcaneonavicular joint (coxa pedis), which is essential for pronation and supination of the foot in its entirety. Conversely, the calcaneocuboid joint function is more discrete, adding flexibility to the foot while providing suspension to the pulley of the peroneus longus tendon [32].

When functioning as a combined unit, the midtarsal joint works to balance the pronatory and supinatory motion initiated by the subtalar joint. When the midtarsal joint unlocks in the pronated subtalar joint, the calcaneocuboid joint functions independently. The cuboid becomes unstable, and the peroneus longus cannot function normally. There is an unopposed function of the tibialis anterior causing supination of the forefoot on the rearfoot at the midtarsal joint. This allows for a loss of medial column stability, because the first ray is no longer plantarflexed [33].

According to Green and Carol [31], midtarsal joint motion occurs in response to the function of the subtalar joint, and planal dominance can be determined with clinical examination in a similar manner to subtalar joint examination. There are two joint axes of the midtarsal joint. The longitudinal axis is oriented 9° from the sagittal plane and 15° from the transverse plane. The oblique axis is oriented 57° from the sagittal plane and 52° from the transverse plane. Thus, the motion around the longitudinal axis is primarily frontal plane motion (inversion-eversion) and the motion around the oblique axis is sagittal plane motion (flexion-extension) and transverse plane motion (abduction-adduction).

Center of rotation of angulation

The CORA is defined as the junction between the mechanical axis and the anatomic axis. The CORA plays a role in the correction of the pediatric flexible flatfoot, because deformities are typically located at the center of rotation of angulation [34]. Although this concept is easily applied to the long bones of the lower extremity and the rearfoot, it becomes more challenging when applied to the foot itself. By the most stringent of definitions, there is no true anatomic axis of the foot, because there are multiple joints that comprise the midfoot and forefoot. Instead of dismissing this principle, however, some aspects of the theory can still be applied to determining the location of the correction.

Because the CORA determines the location of the correction, we can consider the CORA to imply the apex of the deformity. In the long bones of the leg, the CORA has become a proven means of determining the apex of the deformity while considering the most functional correction. In addition, the angular relations and the CORA provide valuable information regarding the magnitude of the deformity. If we assume the CORA to be the apex of the deformity in the foot, we can still accurately determine the optimal and most functional correction of the flexible flatfoot.

Determining the deformity location is dependent on the understanding of some terminology and radiographic measurements:

1. Anatomic axis of the tibia: the middiaphyseal line of the tibia
2. Center of the ankle joint: the center of the talar dome on the anteroposterior (AP) view or the area of the talar dome that is in line with the lateral talar process on the lateral view
3. Ankle joint orientation line: the line drawn along the surface of the distal tibial plafond parallel to the articular surface
4. Angular correction axis (ACA): an imaginary axis in space around which the correction is performed
5. Transverse bisection line (tBL): the transverse bisection line of the angle β created by the proximal and distal axes of bone, which create the CORA (Fig. 1)
6. Longitudinal bisection line (lBL): the longitudinal bisection line of the angle α created by the proximal and distal axes bone; the lBL is always oriented perpendicular to the tBL

There are some angular relations that also need explaining to determine the location of the deformity properly. These angular relations also help to identify the dominant plane of compensation.

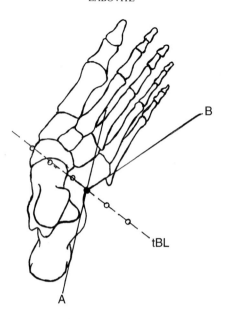

Fig. 1. Line A and line B are drawn adjacent to the lateral surface of the calcaneus and the lateral surface of the cuboid, respectively, comprising the calcaneocuboid angle. The line bisecting the angle is the transverse bisection line, which corresponds to multiple CORAs.

Frontal plane deformity
1. Lateral distal tibial angle: the angle at the junction of the anatomic axis of the tibia and the ankle joint orientation line on the AP radiograph; normal is 89° ± 3° (Fig. 2).
2. Tibial-calcaneal angle: the angle created by the bisection of the anatomic axis of the tibia and the middiaphyseal line of the calcaneus on the rearfoot alignment view or on the long leg calcaneal view; the lines should be parallel, and the calcaneal bisection should be 5 to 10 mm lateral to the anatomic axis of the tibia (Fig. 3).

Sagittal plane deformity
1. Anterior distal tibial angle: the junction between the anatomic axis of the tibia and the ankle joint orientation line on the lateral radiograph; normal is 80° ± 3° (Fig. 4).
2. Talocalcaneal angle: the intersection of the bisection of the talar neck and the plantar surface of the calcaneus on the lateral view; normal is 25° to 45°.
3. Calcaneal inclination angle: the angle created by the junction of the line along the weight-bearing surface and the line drawn along the plantar surface of the calcaneus on the lateral radiograph; normal is 18° to 23°.

4. Talar–first metatarsal angle: the junction between the line bisecting the talar neck and the middiaphyseal line of the first metatarsal on the lateral view; normally these lines are parallel. If the patient is less than 3 years of age, the bisection of the osseous growth center of the talus should bisect the upper third of the cuboid.

Transverse plane deformity
1. Talocalcaneal angle: the bisection of the talar neck and the lateral border of the calcaneus form the talocalcaneal angle on the AP view; normal is 20° to 35° (Fig. 5).
2. Calcaneocuboid angle: the junction between the line drawn parallel to the lateral surface of the calcaneus and the lateral surface of the cuboid; this angle is drawn on the AP radiograph, and it is normally 0° (see Fig. 1).
3. Talar–first metatarsal angle: the intersection of the bisection of the talar neck and the middiaphyseal line of the first metatarsal on the AP radiograph; normal is 0°, because these lines should be parallel.
4. Talonavicular congruity: the articulation of the talonavicular joint is evaluated, and there is typically at least 75% of the talar head articulating with the navicular on the AP view taken in a resting calcaneal stance position.

This terminology provides the surgeon with the means to find the location of the deformity, and thus the optimal location for the correction. When applying this theory

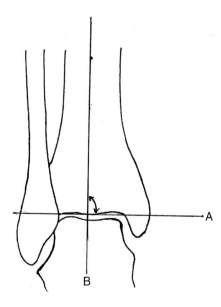

Fig. 2. Line A corresponds to the ankle joint orientation line, and line B corresponds to the anatomic axis of the tibia. The lateral distal tibial angle is located at the junction of these lines.

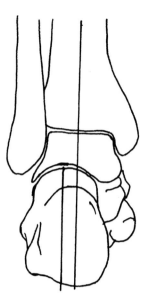

Fig. 3. The anatomic axis of the tibia and the middiaphyseal line of the calcaneus make up the tibial calcaneal angle.

to clinical practice, there are three basic osteotomy principles. First, if the osteotomy is made through the ACA at the CORA, no translation or angulation occurs while achieving the desired correction. Second, if the osteotomy is made at the ACA but not at the CORA, there is translation without angulation. Third, if the osteotomy is made distant to the ACA and the CORA, translation and angulation occur [35,36].

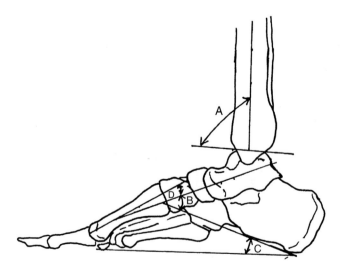

Fig. 4. The lateral view depicts the anterior distal tibial angle (*A*), talocalcaneal angle (*B*), calcaneal inclination angle (*C*), and the talo–first metatarsal angle (*D*).

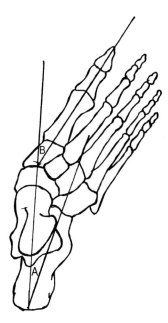

Fig. 5. The AP view of the foot depicts the talocalcaneal angle (*A*) and the talo–first metatarsal angle (*B*).

To achieve the optimal correction without secondary translation or angulation, the osteotomy should be performed at the CORA along the ACA. The proximal and distal axes become linearly aligned when the ACA passes through the CORA along the tBL, however. Thus, there are multiple CORAs in space along the tBL (see Fig. 1) [35].

Multiple apical deformities, such as skewfoot, may occur in the pediatric flatfoot. When applying these principles to the multiapical deformities, performing a single osteotomy or multiple osteotomies can address the deformity. A single osteotomy accounts for the most proximal axis and distal axis to form a resolution CORA, which accounts for the summation of the angular relations. This creates a rectus appearance and function with multiple levels of angulation persistent along the anatomic axis. There may also be some translation along the anatomic axis. When multiple osteotomies are done, they are performed at each true CORA.

The CORA, ACA, and tBL have only accounted for the geometry of the deformity. The clinical parameters, such as an intra-articular location, tendon insertion, or physis, also need to be considered. If the apex of the deformity is located in an area that is not conducive to correction clinically, the osteotomy should be made as close to the CORA as possible. Many times, the translation and angulation created when the osteotomy is made away from the CORA are clinically insignificant. It may be easier to accept the secondary deformity and perform a more desirable osteotomy based on long-term success or familiarity [35].

Algorithm

When considering the biomechanical approach to the correction of the pediatric pes planovalgus, combining the dominant cardinal plane of the deformity and the location of the deformity determines the optimal procedure or procedures. Thus, the procedures chosen should correct the dominant plane of the deformity at the location of the deformity.

While keeping this in mind, surgical correction according to this algorithm (or any other foot or ankle procedures) can only be effective if more proximal causes of the flatfoot have been ruled out. When planning the surgical correction, a thorough musculoskeletal examination should reveal no scoliosis, limb length discrepancy, femoral anteversion, genu valgum, or other proximal forming forces causing the appearance of pathologic flatfoot. Surgical correction of feet with more proximal causes can lead to disasters. For example, a subtalar joint arthroereisis or calcaneal osteotomy on a patient with femoral anteversion or severe tibial torsion can result in a medially rotated arch with respect to the leg [2]. In the adult patient, it has been reported that the surgeon should combine bony realignment and soft tissue procedures because neither alone has adequately corrected the alignment [37]. The surgeon must rule out rigid causes, and they should be addressed outside the scope of this algorithm.

The type of procedure is then selected from the long list of well-established procedures. Table 3 has taken the previous lists of procedures from the historical perspective and reorganized them to address the plane of correction. The soft tissue and osseous procedures are both listed within the table.

When choosing whether a soft tissue procedure or an osseous procedure is warranted, we revert back to the basic principles of flexible versus rigid de-

Table 3
Procedures based on planal dominance

Sagittal plane	Frontal plane	Transverse plane
Kidner procedure	L-shaped osteotomy	Evans osteotomy
Young's tenosuspension	Medial displacement	Calcaneo-cuboid distraction
TAL/Gastrocnemius recession	calcaneal osteotomy	arthrodesis
Spring ligament desmoplasty	Koutsogiannis	Cuboid osteotomy
Cotton osteotomy	Reverse Dwyer	Medial cuneiform osteotomy
Lowman arthrodesis	Gleich	
Miller arthrodesis	Silver	
Hoke arthrodesis	Lord	
	STJ arthroereisis	

Abbreviations: STJ, subtalar joint; Tal, Tendo Achilles lengthening.

formity. Soft tissue procedures can be used in children more frequently than in the adult population, because there is plasticity and the secondary bony changes are unlikely to have occurred in younger children [38]. It is well documented that tendon and ligament procedures deteriorate over time, however, with eventual recurrence of the condition and the symptoms [24]. Osseous procedures are less likely to have recurrent deformities even in children, despite the aforementioned benefits in children. This may necessitate a more aggressive approach as the child ages, with more procedure combinations and a tendency toward more osseous procedures as the child ages [28]. Osseous procedures are also more likely to be successful in the patient with ligamentous laxity as the cause of the pes planovalgus, because the locking mechanism of the subtalar joint may not function [2]. Children aged 6 to 8 years or younger respond well to soft tissue distraction alone when dealing with Ilizarov applications in foot surgery [38]. In the subsequent algorithms, the younger child refers to a child 6 to 8 years of age or younger.

The surgeon must also consider the osseous development of the child. Before surgical correction, an open physis must be accounted for, because there is an increased risk of physeal injury. If the location of the deformity is in close proximity to an open physis, an alternative procedure must be done to prevent injury to the physis. Secondary adaptive changes must also be addressed. If the degenerative changes are noted as a response to the main deforming force, they are typically not found at the location of the deformity. These secondary changes should be addressed in addition to the location of the deformity. Fortunately, this is usually not a factor in the flexible flatfoot of children. It is more prominent in adult flexible pes planovalgus or in rigid pediatric cases. An arthrodesis procedure in a child should only be attempted as a salvage attempt. Arthrodesis procedures have been shown to cause early degenerative changes to the neighboring joints, which is not desirable in a child [1,24].

As mentioned previously, the age of the patient also affects the procedure(s) of choice. Surgical correction of the flexible flatfoot has been recommended in children as young as 2 to 3 years old so as to prevent adaptive changes from occurring [39]. Others have suggested waiting until the child is 8 to 12 years old or after the arch fully develops, because adaptive changes in the joints typically have not occurred [24]. The Podiatry Institute has advocated a trend toward more osseous procedures as the child ages. At the age of 3 to 6 years, the recommended techniques are tendo-Achilles lengthening, Young's tenosuspension, spring ligament desmoplasty, the Kidner procedure, and tibialis anterior tenodesis [28].

The procedures in the algorithm must be performed from the rearfoot to the forefoot. The rearfoot procedures should be performed first to re-establish the proper alignment of the rearfoot to the leg. By realigning the rearfoot first, the surgeon can obtain a neutral position of the subtalar joint, allowing for a maximally pronated and locked midtarsal joint. This stabilizes the lateral column and provides a true forefoot-to-rearfoot relation. The forefoot procedures can be planned before surgery, and they do not have to be determined during surgery after obtaining the neutral subtalar joint position. Radiographs of the subtalar joint in a neutral position before surgery simulate the forefoot-to-rearfoot position. In addition, clinical examination of the rearfoot-to-leg and forefoot-to-rearfoot relations can be observed with the subtalar joint in a neutral position. One can also evaluate the position in a weight-bearing patient with the subtalar joint in a neutral position.

The author has designed the algorithm to guide the surgeon to the procedure(s) of choice. In the algorithm, the procedures are dependent on the dominant plane of deformity and the CORA. The surgical procedures outlined below are designed to correct the dominant plane of compensation at the CORA while taking into account the flexibility of the pes planovalgus deformity. Alternative procedures can replace those in the algorithm as long as they correct the dominant plane at the apex of the deformity.

If the transverse plane is the dominant compensatory plane, the procedure should be selected from the transverse plane procedures at the location closest to the apex of deformity or along the transverse bisection line (Fig. 6). This is likely to involve an Evans procedure, because it is close to the midtarsal joint, which is frequently the main location of a transverse plane deformity. A posterior calcaneal osteotomy can also be selected if the long leg axial radiograph reveals a significant rearfoot valgus, indicating subtalar joint and midtarsal joint instability [40]. The exception is the gastrocnemius recession or Tendo Achilles lengthening (TAL), one of which is to be done if the calcaneal inclination angle is low and the Silverskiöld test clinically reveals an equinus deformity, because the Evans procedure can exaggerate an equinus deformity [22]. As mentioned previously, the amount of midfoot correction obtained with the Evans procedure is debatable. Although some studies have demonstrated lengthening of the lateral column exclusively [24], Dockery [11] claims that additional procedure(s) should be done to help stabilize the medial column sag. Adjunctive procedures have been reported, such as a Young's tenosuspension, split tibialis anterior tendon transfer, talonavicular plication, and tendo-Achilles lengthening [3,6,41]. In the older child, a cuneiform osteotomy or midfoot arthrodesis at the site of the fault can be done [3,4,30].

When the dominant compensatory plane is the frontal plane, a posterior calcaneal osteotomy should be the initial procedure, because it displaces the Achilles tendon insertion medially, eliminating the valgus moment arm of the Achilles tendon. On realigning the rearfoot to the leg, the true forefoot-to-rearfoot alignment should be evident. Again, a double calcaneal osteotomy may be necessary. Any equinus noted clinically can be addressed with a gastrocnemius recession or tendo-Achilles lengthening. Because equinus is usually an adaptive response to prolonged maximal pronation in the frontal plane, a slight superior angle to the posterior calcaneal osteotomy allows for superior migration of the tuberosity with lateral displacement. This superior displacement can be enough correction in mild equinus. If the surgeon observes a medial column fault, a soft tissue procedure in the younger child or a plantarflexory osteotomy in the older child should be performed. An arthrodesis of the medial column can be done on some children depending on the skeletal age of the patient (Fig. 7).

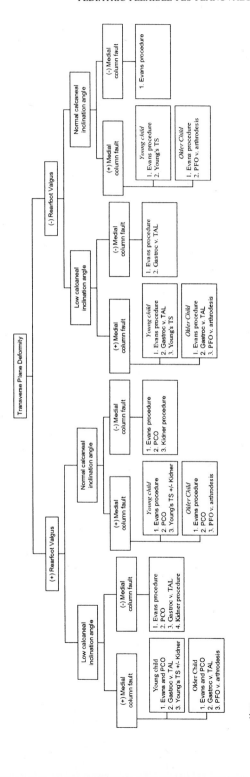

Fig. 6. The algorithm for the transverse plane dominant flatfoot.

Key:
1. PCO = Posterior Calcaneal Osteotomy
2. Gastroc = Gastrocnemius recession
3. Young's TS = Young's tenosuspension
4. PFO = Plantarflexory Osteotomy
** All PFO vs. arthrodesis have the procedure done at the apex of the deformity

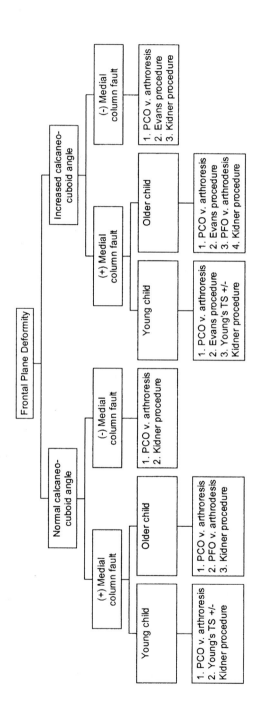

Fig. 7. The algorithm for the frontal plane dominant flatfoot.

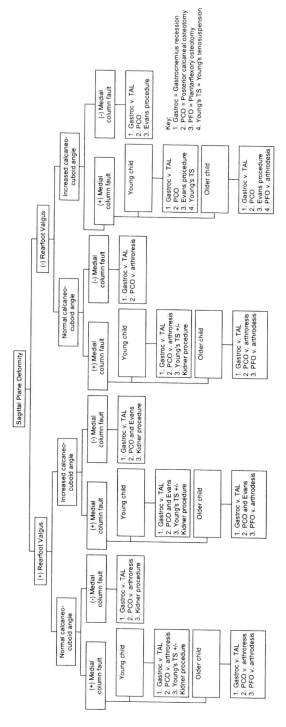

Fig. 8. The algorithm for the sagittal plane dominant flatfoot.

The sagittal plane deformity involves a gastrocnemius recession or tendo-Achilles lengthening depending on the results of the Silverskiöld test. A posterior calcaneal osteotomy should also be performed if the long leg axial radiograph reveals a significant rearfoot valgus. This procedure can be substituted for a subtalar joint arthroereisis. An Evans procedure is added if there is a significantly increased calcaneocuboid angle. A medial column fault necessitates correction at the apex of the deformity, with soft tissue or osseous correction depending on the age of the patient (Fig. 8).

Summary

The author has presented an alternative approach to the pediatric flexible pes planovalgus patient. Hopefully, this algorithm can serve as a guide and not as a rule. It is meant to serve the foot and ankle surgeon as a means of eliminating the arbitrary assignment of a flatfoot to procedures. Instead, the algorithm assigns procedures to a type of flatfoot. The specific procedures listed are a guide to reduce our failures while continually improving our successes.

Acknowledgments

The author thanks Steve Wan, DPM, for editorial assistance and numerous and ongoing discussions regarding surgical biomechanics.

References

[1] Staheli L. Evaluation of planovalgus foot deformities with special reference to the natural history. J Am Podiatr Med Assoc 1987;77(1):2–6.
[2] Pressman M. Biomechanics and surgical criteria for flexible pes valgus. J Am Podiatr Med Assoc 1982;77(1):7–13.
[3] Mosca VS. Calcaneal lengthening for valgus deformity of the hindfoot. J Bone Joint Surg Am 1995;77:500–12.
[4] Anderson AF, Fowler SB. Anterior calcaneal osteotomy for symptomatic juvenile pes planus. Foot Ankle Int 1984;4(5):274–83.
[5] Phillips GE. A review of elongation of os calcis for flat feet. J Bone Joint Surg Br 1983;65(1): 15–8.
[6] Cohen-Sobel E, Giorgini R, Velez Z. Combined technique for surgical correction of pediatric severe flexible flatfoot. J Foot Ankle Surg 1995;34(2):183–94.
[7] Lord JP. Correction of extreme flatfoot. Value of osteotomy of os calcis and inward displacement of posterior fragment. JAMA 1923;81:1502.
[8] Koutsogiannis E. Treatment of hypermobile flat foot by displacement osteotomy of the calcaneus. J Bone Joint Surg Br 1971;53:96–100.
[9] Grumbine NA, Cachia VV, Chin ES, et al. Calcaneal "L" osteotomy: a retrospective study. J Foot Surg 1991;30(4):325–35.
[10] Dwyer FC. Osteotomy of the calcaneum for pes cavus. J Bone Joint Surg Br 1959;41:80–6.

[11] Dockery GL. Surgical treatment of the symptomatic juvenile flatfoot condition. Clin Podiatr Med Surg 1987;4(1):99–117.

[12] Langford JH, Bozof H, Horowitz BD. Subtalar arthroereisis. Clin Podiatr Med Surg 1987; 4(1):153–61.

[13] Lundeen RO. The Smith STA-Peg operation for hypermobile pes planovalgus in children. J Am Podiatr Med Assoc 1985;75(4):177–83.

[14] Nelson SC, Haycock DM, Little ER. Flexible flatfoot treatment with arthroereisis: radiographic improvement and child health survey analysis. J Foot Ankle Surg 2004;43(3):144–55.

[15] Tompkins MH, Nigro JS, Mendicino S. The Smith STA-Peg: a 7-year retrospective study. J Foot Ankle Surg 1993;32(1):27–33.

[16] Addante JB, Chin MW, Loomis JC, et al. Subtalar joint arthroereisis with SILASTIC silicone sphere: a retrospective study. J Foot Surg 1992;31(1):47–51.

[17] Butte FL. Navicular-cuneiform arthrodesis for flat-foot: an end-result study. J Bone Joint Surg [Am] 1937;19:496–502.

[18] Seymour N. The late results of the naviculo-cuneiform fusion. J Bone Joint Surg Br 1967;49(3): 558–9.

[19] Crego Jr CH, Ford LT. An end-result study of various operative procedures for correcting flat feet in children. J Bone Joint Surg Am 1952;34:183–95.

[20] Fraser RK, Menelaus MB, Williams PF, et al. The Miller procedure for mobile flat feet. J Bone Joint Surg Br 1995;77:396–9.

[21] Chi TD, Toolan BC, Sangeorzan BJ, et al. The lateral column lengthening and medial column stabilization procedures. Clin Orthop 1999;365:81–90.

[22] Mahan KT, McGlamry ED. Evans calcaneal osteotomy for flexible pes valgus deformity. Clin Podiatr Med Surg 1987;4(1):137–51.

[23] Sangeorzan BJ, Mosca V, Hansen Jr ST. Effect of calcaneal lengthening on relationships among the hindfoot, midfoot, and forefoot. Foot Ankle 1993;14(3):136–41.

[24] Roye D, Raimondo R. Surgical treatment of the child's and adolescent's flexible flatfoot. Foot Ankle Clin 1998;3(4):593–608.

[25] Davitt JS, MacWilliams BA, Armstrong PF. Plantar pressure and radiographic changes after distal calcaneal lengthening in children and adolescents. J Pediatr Orthop 2001;21(1):70–5.

[26] Jacobs AM, Oloff LM. Surgical management of forefoot supinatus in flexible flatfoot deformity. J Foot Surg 1984;23:410–9.

[27] Myerson MS, Corrigan J, Thompson F, et al. Tendon transfer combined with calcaneal osteotomy for treatment of posterior tibial tendon insufficiency: a radiological investigation. Foot Ankle Int 1995;16:712–8.

[28] Mahan KT, Flanigan KP. Pathologic pes valgus deformity. In: Banks A, Downey MS, Martin DE, et al, editors. McGlamry's comprehensive textbook of foot and ankle surgery. 3rd edition. Philadelphia: Lippincott Williams & Wilkins; 2001. p. 799–861.

[29] Catanziriti AR, Lee MS, Mendicino RW. Posterior calcaneal displacement osteotomy for adult acquired flatfoot. J Foot Ankle Surg 2000;39(1):2–14.

[30] Dollard MD, Marcinko DE, Lazerson A, et al. The Evans calcaneal osteotomy for correction of flexible flatfoot syndrome. J Foot Surg 1984;23(4):291–301.

[31] Green DR, Carol A. Planal dominance. J Am Podiatr Med Assoc 1984;74(2):98–103.

[32] Klaue K. Chopart injuries. Injury 2004;35(Suppl 2):B64–70.

[33] Root ML, Orien WP, Weed JH. Normal and abnormal function of the foot. Los Angeles (CA): Clinical Biomechanics Corporation; 1977. p. 77.

[34] Paley D. Frontal plane mechanical and anatomic axis planning. In: Herzenberg JE, editor. Principles of deformity correction. New York: Springer; 2002. p. 61–97.

[35] Paley D. Osteotomy concepts and frontal plane realignment. In: Herzenberg JE, editor. Principles of deformity correction. New York: Springer; 2002. p. 99–154.

[36] Lamm B, Paley D. Deformity correction planning for hindfoot, ankle, and lower limb. Clin Podiatr Med Surg 2004;21(3):305–26.

[37] Trnka H, Easley ME, Myerson MS. The role of calcaneal osteotomies for correction of adult flatfoot. Clin Orthop 1999;365:50–64.

[38] Herzenberg J, Paley D. Ilizarov applications in foot and ankle surgery. Adv Orthop Surg 1992; 16(3):162–74.

[39] Smith SD, Millar EA. Arthroereisis by means of a subtalar polyethylene peg implant for correction of hindfoot pronation in children. Clin Orthop 1983;181:15–23.

[40] Catanzariti AR, Mendicino RW, King GL, et al. Double calcaneal osteotomy: realignment considerations in eight patients. J Am Podiatr Med Assoc 2005;95(1):53–9.

[41] Viegas GV. Reconstruction of the pediatric planovalgus foot by using an Evans calcaneal osteotomy and augmentative medial split tibialis anterior tendon transfer. J Foot Ankle Surg 2003;42(4):199–207.

ELSEVIER
SAUNDERS

Clin Podiatr Med Surg
23 (2006) 77–118

CLINICS IN
PODIATRIC
MEDICINE AND
SURGERY

Difficult and Controversial Pediatric Cases: A Roundtable on Conservative and Surgical Management

Jonathan M. Labovitz, DPM[a], Marc A. Benard, DPM[b],
Edwin J. Harris, DPM[c,d,*], Harold D. Schoenhaus, DPM[e]

[a]3400 Lomita Blvd., #4093, Torrance, CA 90505, USA
[b]22910 Crenshaw Blvd., #B, Torrance, CA 90505, USA
[c]Department of Orthopaedic Surgery, Stritch School of Medicine, Loyola University Medical Center,
2160 S. 1st Avenue, Maywood, IL 60153, USA
[d]Dr. William M. Scholl College of Podiatric Medicine, Rosalind Franklin University of Health Sciences,
3333 Green Bay Road, North Chicago, IL 60064, USA
[e]Temple University School of Podiatric Medicine, Eighth at Race Street,
Philadelphia, PA 19107, USA

Pediatric clinical management is highly specialized and demands a level of skill and experience that may not be available to most practitioners. Problems are complex and often complicated by other medical issues that dictate limitations on therapeutic options. The presence of open physes limits some therapeutic interventions. Imaging of the immature skeleton is difficult to interpret. The surgeon has to deal with the parents in addition to the child. After therapeutic interventions are initiated, they are irreversible.

A number of questions need to be answered. Can pediatric deformities ever be fully corrected and made normal? Can you justify nonoperative therapy that, in your best professional opinion, is unlikely to work just so you can say you tried everything first? When is "conservative" treatment "radical" and inappropriate? What are the roles of procedures designed to improve and stabilize deformity but not fully correct it? What are the roles in pediatrics for procedures that are clearly salvage techniques in adults? Is joint fusion a viable option in children and

* Corresponding author. Department of Orthopaedic Surgery, Stritch School of Medicine, Loyola University Medical Center, 2160 S. 1st Avenue, Maywood, IL 60153.
  E-mail address: eharrisdpm@aol.com (E.J. Harris).

0891-8422/06/$ – see front matter © 2006 Elsevier Inc. All rights reserved.
doi:10.1016/j.cpm.2005.10.010
podiatric.theclinics.com

adolescents? Is there only one clear-cut answer or are there several equally attractive approaches?

Appropriate diagnosis and successful clinical management depend on the experience and skill of the surgeon. This roundtable discussion, moderated by Jonathan Labovitz, focuses on seven difficult cases and presents the views of three experienced and skilled experts in the field in an attempt to provide personal insights and experiences to help answer these questions.

Case 1—decision making for juvenile hallux abductovalgus

Chief complaint

A 10-year-old girl complains of pain in both feet while wearing shoes. She notices pain especially with athletics and dancing. She rates her pain as 4/10 on a visual analog scale.

The family has noticed lateral deviation of both great toes for several years. They are convinced that the problem is worsening. In addition, there is a strong family history of hallux valgus deformity on the father's side.

Pertinent history

There is no significant history.

Physical findings

Both great toes are laterally deviated. The left underlaps the second toe (Fig. 1A). Hallux dorsiflexion is 50° bilaterally. Subtalar range of motion is 32° of inversion and 10° of eversion on both sides. Ankle dorsiflexion with the knee extended is 10° bilaterally and 15° with the knees flexed. There are no proximal limb deformities and the patient is neurologically intact.

Table 1 displays values derived from radiographs taken at the patient's first visit (see Fig. 1B–E) and those from radiographs taken at another institution 6 months before.

Question 1

What treatment options are available for this child?

Benard

At this juncture, given the progression, I lean strongly toward surgical correction. I presume that underlying neurologic disorders have been accurately assessed and ruled out. I note that the subtalar range of motion is high, which suggests ligamentous laxity. In the clinical photograph, there is prominence of the tibialis anterior tendons at the anterior ankles in bilateral static stance that would not normally be present if the child is positioned in relaxed stance. This finding suggests compensatory firing to maintain medial arch height due to musculoskeletal instability and may be due to ligamentous laxity, midtarsal instability, hyperpronation of the rearfoot, or paresis of the tibialis posterior muscles. The splayed appearance of the firth metatarsals on radiograph further suggests ligamentous laxity.

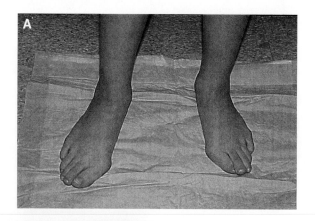

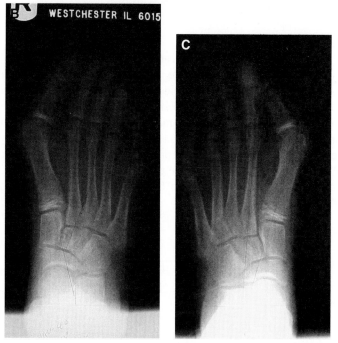

Fig. 1. Case 1—juvenile hallux abductovalgus. (*A*) Clinical photograph. (*B, C*) Anteroposterior radiographs. (*D, E*) Lateral radiographs.

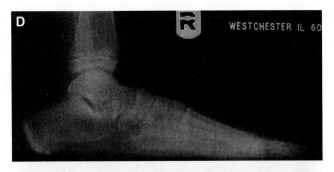

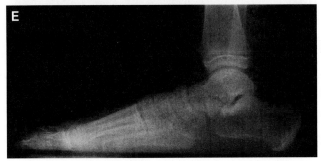

Fig. 1 (*continued*).

Schoenhaus

Treatment options fall under the categories of conservative and surgical management of her deformities. Conservative management of juvenile hallux abductovalgus is limited to bunion shields, wider shoe gear, and orthoses. These devices may provide symptomatic relief. Adolescents may be uncomfortable using some of these devices and they may be viewed as unattractive. Orthotic management may be the most helpful in reducing symptoms until surgery can be performed. They work by controlling pronation, and they may reduce hypermobility of the medial column. Despite the patient's age, surgical management can be considered. The presence of a bunion deformity in the juvenile is a

Table 1
Values derived from radiographs in case 1

	Intermetatarsal angle	Hallux abductus angle	Metatarsus adductus angle
Radiographs at first visit			
Right	13°	40°	20°
Left	16°	45°	24°
Radiographs 6 mo previous			
Right	13°	28°	20°
Left	13°	40°	24°

significant issue. Progression of the deformity can have psychologic and physical sequela and often leads the child and family to consider surgery.

Harris

Nonoperative treatment is the best initial option at this age; however, the parents note progression of what is already a substantial and challenging deformity. The risk of recurrence of the deformity after surgery is high, but additional worsening would make correction even more difficult than it would be at this time. Worsening of the condition outweighs the risk of recurrence. Orthotic control is an option, but there are no data to support the contention that this type of treatment predictably modifies the natural history of the condition. On the other hand, orthotic therapy has no risks, morbidity, or other downsides (except for cost). If this is tried, some realistic end points must be established so that the child does not get caught in the orthosis loop long after the decision to operate should have been made.

Question 2

What factors influence your decision to surgically intervene in a child?

Benard

I consider the severity of symptoms, progression of the deformity, familial predisposition, and extent of hallux abductus when I make that decision.

Schoenhaus

The decision to surgically intervene should not be made lightly. The surgeon has to evaluate the wants of the child and the parents. Although the parents have the ultimate decision (they consent for the child), it must be clear that the child desires correction of the deformity. It is important to assess the degree of pain. The goals of surgery are to reduce pain, improve function at the first meta-tarsophalangeal joint, and stop (or decrease) the progression of the deformity. Adaptive contracture of the first metatarsophalangeal joint, additional deformities (hammertoes), and failure of conservative therapy influence the decision to surgically intervene in a child.

Harris

Rapid progression is an important influencing factor. I also pay attention to the wants of the child and the parents. The impact of the deformity on the child's daily activities is also important. Pain can interfere with the fun things that a child likes to do. Pain can limit participation in sports, dance, and gymnastics. I also suggest studying the child's affect carefully. At this age, surgery may seem like a game. The reality of it does not sink in until the procedure is about to start. Along the same lines, procedures of this type require a high degree of cooperation on the part of the child and the parents. When started, there is no turning back. Failure to comply with the postoperative plan will undo the best surgical technique. The expectations of the child and family must be realistic and attainable. Children at this age are very body-image conscious. They need to know that there are swaps. There will be surgical scars and pain. They may have to submit to some indignities. They will need help with bathing and bathroom functions for a part of the convalescence. There may be some transient or permanent loss of motion. Absolute perfection and "normal" are usually not attainable.

Question 3

What procedures would you consider for this case?

Benard

Before deciding on a choice of procedures, I would need more information— in particular, the frontal plane relationship of the forefoot to rearfoot, the stability of the midtarsal joint with the subtalar joint in neutral position, the axial orientation of the subtalar and midtarsal joints, the position of the tendo-Achilles relative to the posterior leg in bilateral static stance and during gait in midstance and propulsion, and the integrity of the medial column during propulsion.

The degree of ankle joint dorsiflexion in this patient, although acceptable for an adult, is low for a 10-year-old. It suggests compensatory pronation at the subtalar joint with instability of the midtarsal joint.

My surgical approach would include an opening cuneiform osteotomy with autograft or allograft, along with a McBride procedure with or without a Reverdin procedure. I prefer working at the cuneiform level and fashioning a biplane graft that abducts and plantarflexes the first metatarsal. If, as I suspect, pronatory compensation is occurring at the subtalar joint along with significant midtarsal instability, then an opening Evans procedure with autograft or allograft would be included. At that point, I would reassess the ankle joint dorsiflexion on the operating table. If residual gastrocnemius or gastrosoleus equinus is present, then I would perform a gastrocnemius recession or a percutaneous tendo-Achilles lengthening.

Schoenhaus

A number of procedures could be considered and selected by evaluating the clinical and radiographic data. The true intermetatarsal angle must first be computed, which is the intermetatarsal angle plus the metatarsus adductus angle minus 15. The patient's true intermetatarsal angle is 18° on the right and 25° on the left. With such a severe bunion deformity (normal intermetatarsal angle is 8° or less), a proximal first metatarsal osteotomy or a metatarsocuneiform arthrodesis are the two procedures indicated for this patient. Closing base wedge osteotomy, crescentic osteotomy, and opening base wedge osteotomy could be considered. This patient does not have a significant shortening of the first metatarsal, so the crescentic closing base wedge osteotomy would be better than the opening wedge. The other surgical consideration would be first metatarsocuneiform fusion. This procedure would probably not be indicated for this patient because of the open first metatarsal epiphyseal plate. Its presence is not an absolute contraindication, but caution should be taken. Shortening with this procedure may be compensated for with a bone graft.

Harris

The intermetatarsal angle is so large that it cannot be reduced enough by any lateral head displacement procedure. Osteotomy at the base is a better option. I would recommend avoiding fusion of the first metatarsocuneiform joint because of the open physis. Although the plate might survive, closure at this age will have a bad effect on first metatarsal length. I would prefer to correct the intermetatarsal angle on the proximal side of the first metatarsal with an open-up osteotomy of the first cuneiform. Generous lateral release of the first metatarsophalangeal joint soft tissues is also important. Because of the patient's age, it is important to spare the metatarsal head as much as possible so that there will be something to salvage later if the deformity recurs.

Question 4

What would be your postoperative follow-up?

Benard

I tend toward conservative management to protect the surgery from the child. If all of the procedures I mentioned previously were performed (including of gastrocnemius or tendo-Achilles work), then I would place the child in a long leg cast, with non–weight bearing, for 4 weeks, then convert to a short-leg non–weight-bearing cast for an additional 4 weeks, and finally convert to a short-leg weight-bearing cast for 2 to 3 weeks. These time frames are dependent on radiographic evidence of graft incorporation. Afterward, I favor a formal program of physical therapy to restore muscle strength and to normalize gait.

Schoenhaus

Postoperative follow-up would include 6 to 8 weeks of non–weight bearing in a below-knee cast with crutches. After 2 weeks, the cast would be removed for suture removal. A cast would be reapplied. Postoperative radiographs should be taken at 1 week, 3 weeks, between the fourth and sixth week, again at 8 weeks, and every month after that for a year. There will be calf atrophy and stiffness of the ankle and foot joints following cast removal after 6 to 8 weeks. Physical therapy for 4 to 6 weeks can be started so long as the radiographs demonstrate healing at the osteotomy sites. Follow-up should be yearly until age 18 years.

Harris

Because of the age of this child, I would follow my surgery with cast immobilization. Before surgery, she would need crutch training in non–weight bearing on the operated side. I would keep her non–weight bearing for 4 to 6 weeks, depending on the appearance of the radiographs. I would use absorbable sutures for the skin so that removal would not be an issue. I would follow this initial cast therapy with an additional 2 weeks of weight bearing in a cast. After that, physical therapy would be ordered to complete rehabilitation. An additional 2 to 4 months out of sports would probably be appropriate. I would follow her regularly over the next 12 to 18 months.

Question 5

What are the risks for hallux abductovalgus correction in a child of this age?

Benard

Given the choice of the hallux abductovalgus procedure described, the surgical risk is minimized. I prefer to work at the cuneiform level for correction of the intermetatarsal angle because it allows greater latitude for biplanar or triplanar correction while avoiding epiphyseal damage. Although this child appears to have adequate (if not excessive) first metatarsal length, the cuneiform osteotomy also carries the advantage of preservation of length. In my experience, children also respond well to capital osteotomy. Although I prefer this approach, excellent results can also be obtained with first metatarsal osteotomy distal to the epiphysis in the hands of an experienced pediatric surgeon.

Schoenhaus

Risks associated with hallux abductovalgus correction in a child of this age include damage to the epiphysis when performing procedures at the base of the first metatarsal. This damage results in growth arrest. Iatrogenic medial displacement of the sesamoids with hallux varus is another complication. Staking of the first metatarsal head can also lead to hallux varus. With a closing base wedge osteotomy, there is always a risk of first metatarsal elevatus. Numbness, tingling, infection, and recurrence round out the risks.

Harris

Of course, there are the usual risks. Anesthesia is a big parental concern, but in the healthy child, it is an acceptable risk. Infection is a concern in general, but more so in a child because of compliance with common-sense issues with casts. This age group considers itself indestructible. Bad things from soiling or wetting the cast always happen to others, never to them. The same thing can be said for malunion or nonunion. That sort of complication always happens to someone else, never to them. I would consider these risks higher because of the age group. Recurrence of the deformity in children is always a big worry for me and even more of a risk in this child because of the severity of the deformity. Even if the medial column correction is performed in the first cuneiform, there is still worry about the first metatarsal epiphyseal plate, which could be damaged by vascular compromise, compression from first-ray elongation, or by fixation of the osteotomies. I have passed smooth wires across epiphyseal plates on multiple occasions without causing plate closure, but it is still a risk.

Case 2—cavovarus deformity

Chief complaint

A 12-year-old boy has high arches that were first noted when his basketball coach took him off the team because of concerns that he was unstable and prone to injury. Until that time, there had been no concerns (Fig. 2A–D).

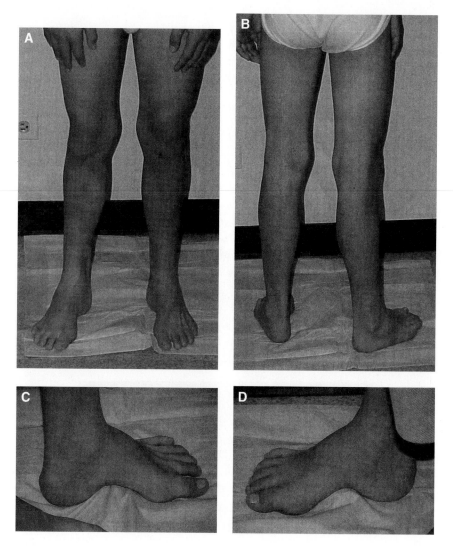

Fig. 2. Case 2—cavovarus deformity. (*A–D*) Clinical photographs. (*E, F*) Anteroposterior radiographs. (*G, H*) Lateral radiographs.

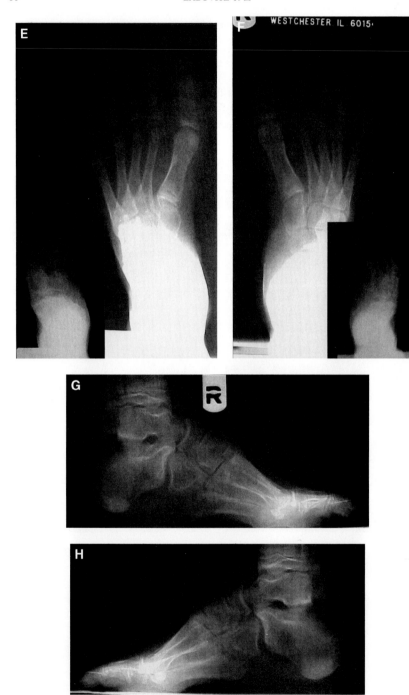

Fig. 2 (*continued*).

Pertinent history

Past medical history is unremarkable. Pregnancy, developmental history, and systems review are noncontributory. Family history has Charcot-Marie-Tooth disease traceable to the maternal great-grandmother. His mother and his 9-year-old brother have high-arched feet.

Physical findings

The patient has a bilateral steppage gait, with difficulty clearing during swing phase as he attempts a heel-to-toe gait. Biomechanical data are shown in Table 2. Neurologic examination reveals muscle strengths are 5/5, except for bilateral 3+/5 anterolateral leg compartments. Deep tendon reflexes are absent in the upper and lower extremities. Sensory examination reveals that sharp/dull is intact on both sides; vibratory sensation is decreased in the upper and lower extremities. Anteroposterior radiographs show adduction of the forefoot with very narrow anteroposterior talocalcaneal angles (see Fig. 2E, F). Lateral radiographs show a horizontal talus, high calcaneal inclination angle, and plantarflexed medial column bilaterally (see Fig. 2G, H).

Question 1

Despite the obvious, what additional diagnoses would you include in the differential?

Benard

The presentation is strongly suggestive for Charcot-Marie-Tooth disease. The most frequent subtype encountered is of the demyelinating variety, often type 1A or 1B. I suppose one might consider alternative hereditary motor-sensory conditions of the axonal variety such as type 2A through type 2E. Although other conditions might explain the presence of progressive cavus deformity (neurofibromatosis or cerebral palsy, to name two), they can easily be eliminated

Table 2
Biomechanical data for case 2

Examination	Right	Left
Subtalar ROM inversion/eversion	25°/12°	25°/12°
Ankle ROM knee extended	+2°	+5°
Ankle ROM knee flexed	+5°	+10°
Tibial torsion	Out 30°	Out 25°
Popliteal angle	60°	60°
Hip ROM extended in/out	10°/50°	25°/30°
Hip ROM flexed in/out	45°/50°	35°/50°

Abbreviation: ROM, range of motion.

through physical examination and clinical presentation. Cerebral palsy affecting primarily the extrapyramidal system would result in contracture at a much earlier age. Manual reduction of the equinus would characteristically be spongy, slowly returning to an equinus condition when manual resistance is removed. Deep tendon reflexes would also be present. Neurofibromatosis could easily present this early; however, this is not consistent with a bilaterally symmetric presentation. In my experience, it is more apt to present as equinovarus than as calcaneocavus.

Schoenhaus

In addition to Charcot-Marie-Tooth disease, I would consider Roussy-Lévy syndrome, Friedreich's ataxia, Dejerene-Sottas disease, and spinal dysraphisms.

Harris

My fellow panel members have considered all of the differentials. I would add that careful inspection of the back may show some skin changes that may indicate cord pathology. Tethering of the cord can occur without any outward physical findings. Foot deformity, particularly cavus deformity, is frequently the first and only finding. Questioning about bowel and bladder function is important. An MRI of the cord is in order if there is no obvious diagnosis.

Question 2

What testing and imaging would you order to clarify the diagnosis?

Benard

Nerve conduction velocity and electromyography are definitely indicated. Nerve and muscle biopsy are standard practice. The subtypes of Charcot-Marie-Tooth disease produce a variety of clinical patterns defined by the severity of involvement, age at onset, and ranges of nerve conduction velocities. Genetic markers have been identified for the specific subtypes. For the treating podiatrist, the clinical significance is that all cavus feet are not alike, and a thorough history and physical examination must be conducted. A hereditary sensory-motor or motor neuropathy must always be suspected in a child this age with this level of deformity, even when a strong familial pattern is not present.

Imaging studies are not needed to clarify my diagnosis, but I prefer medial radiographs to lateral radiographs in cavus feet. As can be seen in the lateral radiographs (see Fig. 2G, H), the shape of the foot obligates the ankle mortise to be externally rotated when the medial border of the foot is placed against the radiographic plate. This rotation results in a posteriorly positioned fibula and in external rotation of the talus. The talus is therefore artificially foreshortened. The trochlear surface and the ankle joint articulation are not well visualized. In less mature feet, when the ossification of the medial and lateral portions of the trochlear surface are less well defined, rotation may lead to a misdiagnosis of talar flattening when none is truly present.

Schoenhaus

Careful neurologic examination should include evaluation of deep tendon reflexes, qualitative sensory analysis, and manual muscle testing. Electromyographic and nerve conduction velocity studies give valuable information. Muscle and nerve biopsy may be indicated on rare occasions. Specific genetic testing is available for many of these problems. Limb MRI can evaluate muscle distribution and size.

Harris

A careful and complete neurologic examination is the first step. Associated patterns of weakness can help narrow down the pathology to one of several groups. Sensory examination should include vibratory and positional sense. Presence or absence of deep tendon reflexes helps to further narrow down the differential. Electromyography and nerve conduction velocities should be ordered when the examiner has a strong suspicion about the pathophysiology. These tests rarely make the diagnosis when they are randomly ordered, and the result of inappropriate testing may lead to incorrect assumptions. MRI of the brain and spinal cord should be considered when there is no obvious diagnosis.

Question 3

Motor nerve conduction velocity averages 12 m/s, and DNA studies confirm Charcot-Marie-Tooth disease type 1A. What nonoperative treatment would you attempt?

Benard

Several reasonable choices exist at this point. Stock or custom-molded ankle-foot orthoses (AFOs) would stabilize the frontal and sagittal planes and assist with ground clearance and lateral instability. Another alternative is a Richie-type AFO because muscle strength in the anterior and lateral groups is still graded at +3/5 (antigravity strength).

Schoenhaus

AFOs would be useful. Physical therapy would also be indicated.

Harris

Steppage gait suggests that there are problems clearing the swing limb. An AFO would convert the patient back to a heel-toe pattern for the short-term. I do not expect that the patient would continue to respond because of the natural history of this disease. Progressive equinus would eventually make it impossible to use an AFO, and the patient already has a limited range and clearing difficulties during swing. Physical therapy might slow down the development of equinovarus contracture.

Question 4

Over a 6-month period, the deformities are worsening. What would be your surgical goals?

Benard

The overall goal would be to produce a stable platform in the presence of a progressive neurologic pathology that results in structural and functional imbalance in the foot over time. Ultimately, most of these patients require arthrodesing procedures such as triple arthrodesis due to the dynamic imbalance in muscle function brought on by progressive paresis in the anterior, lateral, and intrinsic muscle groups. The clinical course varies case by case, so each patient must be assessed individually. In slowly progressive cases, it may be possible to realign the foot through osteotomy with or without tendon transfer rather than arthrodesis; however, the patient and parents need to be aware that the dynamic nature of the disease may require multiple surgeries.

Schoenhaus

My goals would be to reduce fixed deformity and to restore muscle balance through tendon transfer. An important goal would be to prevent recurrence of the deformity by basing treatment on patient age, progression of the deformity, degree of deformity, and the deforming forces operating.

Harris

At this age, the first goal would be to prevent progression of the deformity. Tibialis posterior tends to be the healthiest of the muscles but becomes the deforming force. It needs to be neutralized. The second goal would be to correct as many of the static deformities as possible. These static deformities include plantar flexion of all or part of the medial column, fixed or flexible inversion of the calcaneus, ankle equinus, and clawing of the toes.

Question 5

What surgical procedures would you consider?

Benard

Given the clinical history of rapid progression, I would perform triple arthrodesis, with angulatory correction in all three planes of deformity. In my experience, ankle block and flat-topped talus are rarely present. Therefore, osseous work would be restricted to structures below the ankle. This 12-year-old has sufficient osseous development to perform the procedure. Typically, hammertoes are present, and when they are flexible (as they usually are in this age bracket), they are treated with tenotomy and pinning. After the postoperative period is complete, I would maintain the child in an AFO until the distal tibial epiphysis is closed and longitudinal growth is completed. Then, depending on the severity of the anterior group paresis, I would typically convert the dysfunctional anterior and lateral muscle-tendon complexes into suspensory ligaments to keep the foot at 90° to the leg. If needed, I would perform ankle arthrodesis as a last resort. The tibialis anterior, extensor hallucis longus, and extensor digitorum longus tendons would be tacked to the tibia at their myotendinous junctions. The peroneus brevis tendon would be sectioned at its myotendinous junction, rerouted into the anterior compartment, and likewise tacked into the tibia. Distally, digital arthrodesis would be performed as required, and the extensor tendon slips tacked to the metatarsal necks.

I would like to comment on what I would not do. Tendo-Achilles lengthening should be avoided. The limitation of ankle joint dorsiflexion in calcaneocavus feet is the result of the plantarflexed forefoot-to-rearfoot relationship. This condition is called pseudoequinus. These patients already display horizontal positioning of the talus, on which tendo-Achilles lengthening would have no corrective effect. The high calcaneal inclination angle in stance further indicates that a soft tissue equinus is not present. The only effect that tendo-Achilles lengthening in this foot type produces is further dynamic imbalance between the plantar intrinsic muscles and the already-weak anterior group, resulting in progression of the calcaneocavus.

Schoenhaus

I would perform a triple arthrodesis and possibly a subtalar joint valgus wedge to avoid a Dwyer osteotomy. The triple arthrodesis would help decrease forefoot equinus, calcaneal varus, and forefoot valgus. The patient would need a dorsiflexory first-ray osteotomy. A plantar release would be necessary, and tibialis posterior would need lengthening or transfer. The patient may need peroneus longus tenotomy with tenodesis to peroneus brevis. If the toes are not reducible, he may need proximal interphalangeal joint arthrodesis.

Harris

I would try to avoid triple arthrodesis because many patients who have Charcot-Marie-Tooth disease have sensory neuropathy, which could put them at risk for neuropathic joint disease in the future. I would also try to avoid triple arthrodesis at this age, even if the child is neurologically intact; however, if the child is unstable because of extreme weakness, this approach needs to be rethought. Given the clinical data of this particular case, I would perform a plantar release, first metatarsal dorsiflexing osteotomy, and transfer of tibialis posterior through the interosseous membrane under the extensor retinaculi to the dorsum of the foot (it functions better if run under the retinaculum). If the tendon is too short to reach its new point of attachment, then subcutaneous routing gives some additional length without seriously compromising function. A lateral displacement calcaneal osteotomy is needed if there is fixed heel varus. If not, then the calcaneus can be left alone. Hammering of the hallux is best managed with a Jones suspension and interphalangeal arthrodesis. Lesser-toe deformity is managed based on severity. Flexor tendon release or transfer may be indicated for mild deformity. More severe deformity requires proximal transfer of extensor digitorum longus and interphalangeal joint fusions.

Case 3—chromosomal abnormality with uncontrollable pronation and ankle valgus deformity

Chief complaint

A 10-year-old boy has chromosomal deletions at several levels that have resulted in cognitive impairment, developmental delay, and hypotonia. He has been ambulating for 8 years but is becoming progressively more pronated. He is currently in bilateral articulated AFOs.

Pertinent history

There are no other medical issues.

Physical findings

There is subtalar range of motion (Table 3). When the heel bisection is in the plane of the tibial axis, the forefoot is supinated about 5° to 6°, with the first metatarsal additionally dorsiflexed (Fig. 3A–C). The gait is a full-flat pattern with knees in extension throughout stance. The patient appears maximally pronated, and there is no calcaneal inversion during gait. The anteroposterior radiograph shows a wide anteroposterior talocalcaneal angle but only 40% of the medial talar head uncovered (see Fig. 3D). The lateral radiograph demonstrates a medial

Table 3
Biomechanical data for case 3

Examination	Right	Left
Subtalar ROM inversion/eversion	20°/25°	25°/20°
Ankle ROM knee extended	+20°	+20°
Ankle ROM knee flexed	+30°	+35°
Tibial torsion	Out 40°	Out 35°
Popliteal angle	25°	25°
Hip ROM extended in/out	40°/40°	40°/40°
Hip ROM flexed in/out	40°/60°	40°/60°

Abbreviation: ROM, range of motion.

column sagittal fault at the talonavicular joint (see Fig. 3E). The anteroposterior ankle radiograph shows a 13° valgus ankle tilt (see Fig. 3F).

At age 12 years, his parents report steady worsening. They are concerned that he is "falling off his left ankle." New anteroposterior ankle radiographs show that the ankle valgus has increased to 22° (see Fig. 3G).

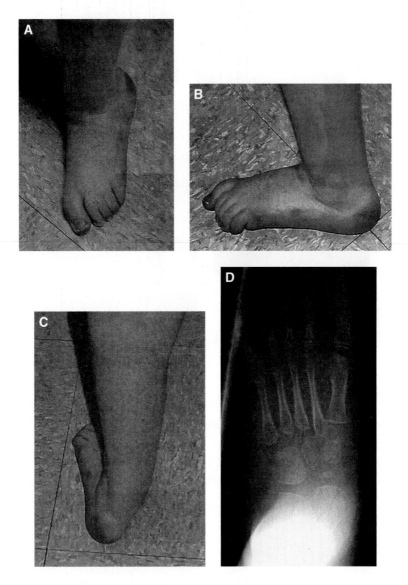

Fig. 3. Case 3—chromosomal abnormality with uncontrollable pronation and ankle valgus deformity. (*A–C*) Clinical photographs. (*D*) Anteroposterior radiograph. (*E*) Lateral radiograph. (*F*) Anteroposterior ankle radiograph. (*G*) Anteroposterior ankle radiograph taken 2 years later.

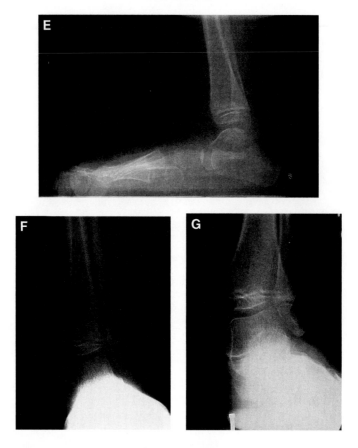

Fig. 3 (*continued*).

Question 1

What nonoperative treatment is there to offer?

Benard
Further bracing, but in a nonarticulated device due to the paresis and progressive ankle valgus.

Schoenhaus
Considering the significant progression of the deformity despite years of AFO use, there are minimal to no conservative options left. The child is too old for casting, and orthoses have failed. Because of the chromosomal abnormality, there may be increased risks for complications that need to be discussed with the parents before the decision for surgical correction is entertained.

Harris

There is a significant deformity on all three planes that is complicated by primary ankle valgus due to the wedged tibial epiphysis. This situation points out the absolute necessity in evaluating the ankle joint in all cases of pronation. Ankle valgus makes it appear pronated and makes bracing very difficult. The skin is already showing signs of intolerance to bracing. If the decision is made to continue orthoses, I seriously doubt that this child could be controlled in anything short of an AFO. Although this form of therapy might buy some time, I do not believe that it will reverse or even slow down the progression of the deformity. This case can only be addressed surgically.

Question 2

What are your surgical goals and objectives?

Benard

As in the other cases, a stable, rectus platform for weight bearing is the main goal. In this case, we are dealing with progressive deformity from paresis and not spasm. Structural stability is the major goal.

Schoenhaus

My goals and objectives are to (1) decrease symptoms with improvement in overall function; (2) improve lower extremity position to prevent potential severe osteoarthritis; (3) address the external tibial rotation, ankle valgus, equinus, pronation, supinatus, and talonavicular malalignment; (4) maintain as much tibial length as possible with an opening wedge osteotomy in preference to a closing wedge osteotomy, keeping in mind that patients with chromosomal abnormalities are usually shorter in stature than average; (5) evaluate limb length preoperatively as a part of surgical planning (at age 12 years, the majority of future growth is most likely at the proximal tibial epiphysis; the distal tibial epiphysis grows more rapidly until 50% of the entire tibial length has been achieved); and (6) evaluate the center of rotation of angulation. In this case, the center of rotation of angulation appears to be near or at the distal tibial epiphysis. Most of the angulation deformity is the result of the epiphyseal wedging. Physeal arrest will most likely be necessary to prevent future reangulation.

Harris

My goals are to (1) stabilize the foot by bringing the calcaneus back to vertical, (2) restore the medial column in the sagittal plane, (3) restore congruency of the talonavicular joint complex, (4) correct the valgus deformity of the distal tibia, and (5) minimize the possibility of recurrence. All of these goals are directed toward making the patient a comfortable and efficient orthosis candidate.

Question 3

What procedures would you perform?

Benard
The child is chronologically age 12 years but appears to be radiographically younger. I would opt for an extra-articular subtalar arthrodesis (Grice procedure), an opening Evans osteotomy with allograft, an opening plantarflexory osteotomy of the medial cuneiform with graft, and stapling of the medial ankle epiphysis. Muscle strength is not available for this patient. I am not confident that adjunctive tendon transfer would be of value. It may also be necessary to perform additional procedures when the child reaches skeletal maturity.

Schoenhaus
I would perform a derotational opening tibial wedge osteotomy using tri-cortical iliac crest bone graft. Fixation requirements may be minimal if the fibula is left intact. Steinmann pins, screws, plates, and external fixators are all options. I would perform a physeal arrest. Tendo-Achilles lengthening is also indicated. After the initial osteotomy is performed, I would re-evaluate and consider arthroereisis with combined Evans and Kutsgiannis osteotomies. A triple arthrodesis may be indicated to control the rearfoot. Medial column arthrodesis with plantarflexing osteotomy is also indicated. Procedures such as triple arthrodesis performed distal to the ankle tend to fail as the primary procedure when there is extensive ankle deformity and rearfoot valgus.

Harris
I would perform Evans osteotomies to lengthen and plantarflex the lateral columns. Given the range of ankle motion, I would not lengthen the tendo-Achilles. I would perform an open-up and plantarflexing first cuneiform osteotomy and fixate it with one or two staples. At that point, the position of the heel needs to be evaluated. If it remains in significant valgus, then a medial displacement osteotomy is indicated. I would handle the ankle valgus with a screw introduced from the tip of the medial malleolus across the physis to produce a temporary epiphyseodesis.

Question 4

What would be your postoperative management?

Benard
Due to the combination of Grice procedure and opening Evans osteotomy, I would maintain the patient non–weight bearing in a short leg cast for 12 weeks

with gradual, protected weight bearing afterward. When the patient is able, I would return him to an AFO molded to his improved foot position and modify it as the ankle valgus reduces with time.

Schoenhaus

I would plan my corrections in stages with follow-up as indicated by the procedure. I would stress that repeat tibial osteotomies might be needed in the future.

Harris

Given the patient's overall status, I would suggest bilateral correction at the same time. Non–weight-bearing cast immobilization would be continued until all osteotomies have united. In the interim, the patient would need a wheelchair for transportation. After the osteotomies are united, I would return him to AFOs for at least a year. Because I have done screw fixation of the medial tibial epiphyseal plates, I would monitor him with serial radiographs. The probability is that the plates will close before the hardware needs to be removed, but overcorrection to ankle varus is a real possibility.

Case 4—pronation unresponsive to orthotic management

Chief complaint

An 11-year-old boy has a history of flatfoot deformity since birth. He was treated with orthoses since age 4 years, but there has not been any improvement. He now has pain in the medial and plantar aspects of both feet with most activities and is giving up on sports.

Pertinent history

Past medical history is unremarkable. Pregnancy, developmental history, and systems review are noncontributory.

Physical findings

The gait shows marked symmetric abduction with maximal heel eversion, no supinatory movement, and prominent talar heads medially. The patient stands in maximal pronation and abduction (Fig. 4A, B). Table 4 shows biomechanical data. The neurologic examination revealed that the patient is neurologically nor-

mal. Anteroposterior radiograph shows extremely wide anteroposterior talocalcaneal angles with beginning subluxation of the talonavicular joints. The forefoot
is abducted. The lateral radiograph shows bilateral sagittal medial column failure
at the talonavicular, cuneonavicular and metatarsocuneiform joints. In addition,
there is metatarsus primus elevatus (see Fig. 4C, D).

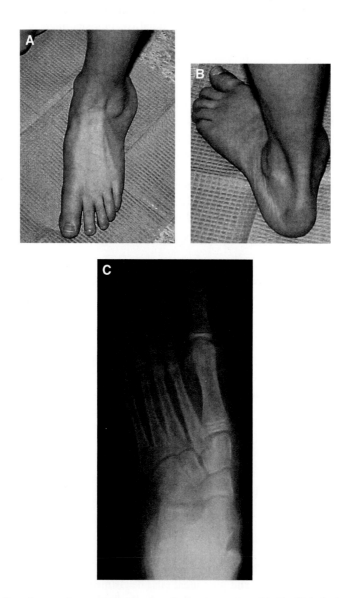

Fig. 4. Case 4—pronation unresponsive to orthotic management. (*A, B*) Clinical photographs.
(*C*) Anteroposterior radiograph. (*D*) Lateral radiograph.

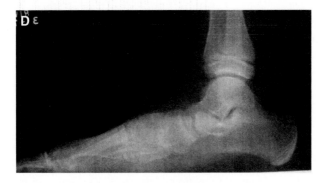

Fig. 4 (*continued*).

Question 1

What nonsurgical therapy is advisable at this point?

Benard

The current orthoses are not described, but the large amount of frontal and transverse plane compensation of the forefoot compels me to consider supramalleolar orthoses for additional control.

Schoenhaus

At this point, considering the age of this patient, conservative treatment is unlikely to be successful. The patient has already failed orthotic management. Adding a night splint to the conservative regimen could also be considered; however, significant improvement should not be expected. Most conservative treatments at this point would be accommodative.

Harris

Nonoperative therapy has failed. I do not see any benefit to continued attempts. Given the severity of the deformity, I think the patient has been a marginal orthosis candidate for a long time. One could argue that orthoses

Table 4
Biomechanical data for case 4

Examination	Right	Left
Subtalar ROM inversion/eversion	30°/15°	25°/12°
Ankle ROM knee extended	+15°	+15°
Ankle ROM knee flexed	+20°	+20°
Tibial torsion	Out 30°	Out 20°
Popliteal angle	30°	30°
Hip ROM extended in/out	25°/35°	25°/35°
Hip ROM flexed in/out	30°/60°	30°/60°

Abbreviation: ROM, range of motion.

might relieve discomfort, but he is already modifying his physical activities to accommodate his deformities. I would abandon nonoperative therapy at this point.

Question 2

What are your surgical goals and objectives for this patient?

Benard

To restore the forefoot-to-hindfoot relationship, stabilize the lateral column, and improve the position and function of the medial column and first ray.

Schoenhaus

The surgical goal for this patient is to achieve a pain-free functional foot and to restore the medial longitudinal arch.

Harris

My goals include producing a reasonably supple pain-free foot in better alignment to allow this child to get on with adolescence. Stopping additional deformity to prevent osteoarthrosis as an adult is also a goal.

Question 3

If surgery is indicated, what is the value of arthroereisis procedures in this case?

Benard

The clinical photograph is not taken from directly posterior; however, it appears that the heel is not excessively everted with subtalar pronation. The tendo-Achilles appears reasonably well centralized relative to the malleoli. In addition, the transverse plane compensation of the midtarsal joint makes the choice of arthroereisis questionable.

Schoenhaus

Subtalar joint arthroereisis would be of value. This procedure limits excessive pronatory motion while preserving varus range of motion. By limiting this motion, the midtarsal joint becomes maximally pronated and locked. In addition to stabilizing the subtalar joint, arthroereisis also exerts a supinatory force on the tarsus during weight bearing. By limiting excessive subtalar pronation, there is significant improvement in the resting calcaneal stance position, a reduction in the talocalcaneal angle, an increase in the calcaneal inclination angle, a decrease in the talar declination angle, and a reduction of talonavicular subluxation. There is an improvement in elevation of the medial arch on weight bearing. The advantages to this procedure include simple technique and indications for the skeletally immature. Results tend to improve with growth.

Harris

The severity of the deformity is great enough that arthroereisis may not be enough to control the deformity, which is triplane pronation with some forefoot supination that is almost certainly fixed. I think I would be considerably more aggressive in my surgical approach.

Question 4

What surgical procedures would you employ in this case?

Benard

Opening Evans osteotomy with autograft; complete peroneus brevis transfer posteriorly to the medial compartment into the navicular or, if possible, the medial cuneiform; and possible plantarflexory osteotomy of the medial cuneiform. Reefing of the spring ligament would be indicated. I would stop there and reassess the foot over time.

Schoenhaus

I would do a subtalar arthroereisis. It appears from the biomechanical data (see Table 4) that the patient has adequate ankle range of motion and is not in need of a tendo-Achilles lengthening or gastrocnemius recession. The arthroereisis alone may be adequate to correct most of the deformity. If more correction of the metatarsus primus elevatus in the sagittal plane is indicated, then I would perform a Cotton osteotomy in the medial cuneiform.

Harris

I would perform an Evans calcaneal osteotomy with a banked bone graft to gain calcaneal length and plantarflex the distal fragment by rotation at the osteotomy site. I would handle the medial column with a plantarflexing osteotomy of the first metatarsal near its base.

Case 5—cerebral palsy with isolated equinus deformity

Chief complaint

A 5-year-old boy carries a diagnosis of spastic diplegia and is a persistent toe-walker.

Pertinent history

The patient is one of triplets delivered at 28 weeks and had a birth weight of 1.4 kg. At 3 days old, he had periventricular leukomalacia following hypoxia and an intracranial bleed. He stayed in pediatric ICU for 3 months. He has been

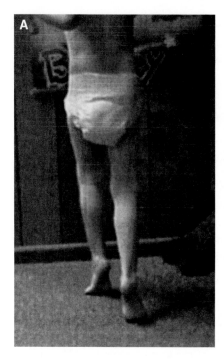
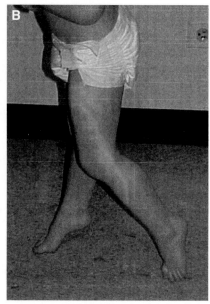

Fig. 5. Case 5—cerebral palsy with isolated equinus deformity. (*A, B*) Clinical photographs.

receiving physical therapy since discharge and is currently in solid-ankle AFOs set at neutral. He no longer stays down on the left side.

Physical findings

The patient's gait is toe-toe bilateral. He can come down to plantigrade on the right, but the left heel is continuously 4 cm off the ground (Fig. 5A, B). Biomechanical data are shown in Table 5. There are no knee or hip flexion contractures and no evidence of hip dysplasia or dislocation. On neurologic

Table 5
Biomechanical data for case 5

Examination	Right	Left
Subtalar ROM inversion/eversion	20°/10°	25°/10°
Ankle ROM knee extended	+5°	−20°
Ankle ROM knee flexed	+10°	−5°
Tibial torsion	Out 20°	Out 14°
Popliteal angle	55°	55°
Hip ROM extended in/out	60°/30°	70°/20°
Hip ROM flexed in/out	60°/45°	70°/40°

Abbreviation: ROM, range of motion.

examination, there is increased tone in all four extremities—more so in the lowers. Upper and lower deep tendon reflexes are +3 bilaterally. Plantar reflex is upgoing with clonus bilaterally. Except for left equinus, the radiographs do not contribute.

Question 1

What nonoperative therapy would you recommend at this time?

Benard

The patient seems like a good candidate for botulinum toxin type A injection into the myotendinous junction of the gastrocnemius. Otherwise, I would opt for tendo-Achilles advancement.

Schoenhaus

Initially, spastic equinus should be treated by the safest techniques, regardless of etiology. The patient is currently being treated with physical therapy and AFOs. Other useful techniques include exercise routines aimed at weakening and stretching the posterior group of muscles while simultaneously strengthening the anterior group. These exercises may be effective for this patient's less contracted extremity. Serial casts can also be used for a reducible deformity and can be followed by bracing and night splints until full skeletal maturity. This patient's deformity, however, is clearly past further conservative management.

Harris

Although the right ankle range of motion is decreased, this side can probably be controlled in an AFO. The left side cannot come anywhere near neutral in any knee position, so an AFO would not help. In my experience, physical therapy alone for patients who have findings similar to this child's right side does not usually result in a useful increase in range of motion. Serial stretching casts have better outcomes, but I believe that serial stretching casts augmented with botulinum toxin type A injections would give the best results. This patient's left deformity is so significant, however, that attempts to brace or cast against this much unyielding equinus would breech the midfoot and damage the talus. He is beyond nonoperative management on that side.

Question 2

Is there any indication for continued physical therapy in this case?

Benard

Physical therapy is effective in the reduction of acquired contractures at the knee and hip, if present, but not particularly good for the ankle. The spastic gastrosoleus complex does not respond well to the dorsiflexory stimulation. A better choice would be partial rhizotomy to reduce the spasm.

Schoenhaus

Physical therapy may improve the patient's gait pattern in the right lower extremity, especially if coupled with biofeedback treatment. Recent studies have shown that children who receive electromyographic feedback training plus conventional exercise therapy have statistically significant improvement in active range of motion and plantarflexor tone compared with control subjects. Physical therapy should definitely be used after surgical correction as an adjunct to decrease the likelihood of recurrence.

Harris

No. At this point, I would not expect any additional gains. Having said that, physical therapy monitoring is appropriate in the short-term to maintain what has already been achieved. In addition, keep in mind that this patient has four-joint level pathology (hip, knee, ankle, and subtalar joint). Even though there are no fixed contractures, alteration in tone and persistent movement patterns can and will produce dynamic contractures.

Question 3

Is there any pharmacologic therapy for this case?

Benard

Botulinum toxin type A is useful.

Schoenhaus

Recent studies have shown that botulinum toxin type A injections into spastic components of the triceps surae may cause weakening and delay the need for surgical treatments in immature patients; however, results are mixed. Logically, this drug would work better in dynamic equinus.

Harris

Botulinum toxin type A injections are useful. I have no personal experience with baclofen and other similar medications.

Question 4

What do you consider when deciding among percutaneous tendo-Achilles lengthening, open tendo-Achilles lengthening, and gastrocnemius recession?

Benard

I am not a fan of these procedures for patients who have upper motor neuron pathology, although I acknowledge that they are widely used. I restrict these procedures to patients who have lower motor neuron pathology or in whom no neurologic pathology is detected. To answer the question, however, in patients who have mild limitation of ankle extension ($-5°$ of dorsiflexion or less with the knee extended) that involves the gastrocnemius and the soleus, percutaneous tendo-Achilles lengthening is my procedure of choice. When greater limitation of dorsiflexion is present with the same etiology, I prefer open tendo-Achilles lengthening, which gives me the option of a more complete posterior release if it is required. Gastrocnemius recession, by medial or lateral resection of the aponeurosis (or both), is used when only the gastrocnemius muscle is determined to be tight. I am aware that isolated soleus recession can also be performed, but I have no personal experience with it.

Schoenhaus

The extent of deformity and the amount of correction desired are the primary considerations. I have concerns about the reliability of outcome with percutaneous tendo-Achilles lengthening in diplegics. In addition, there is the risk of complete transaction with this procedure. Open tendo-Achilles lengthening theoretically reduces the chances of complete transaction, but you are left with a larger incision. Gastrocnemius recessions are known to be more stable and are associated with a slightly lower rate of overlengthening. Gastrocnemius recession may result in less chance for apropulsive gait and calcaneus deformity than tendo-Achilles lengthening.

Harris

The amount of lengthening required is the first consideration. Percutaneous procedures are better when the amount of lengthening is small. For bigger deformities, open tendo-Achilles lengthenings are preferred. An additional benefit to this approach is that a limited posterior release can also be performed. For hemiplegics and diplegics, I prefer gastrocnemius recession. I will do this even if the soleus appears modestly contracted. I have no experience with Murphy advancements in this patient population.

Question 5

What surgical intervention would you choose for this case?

Benard

As described briefly in a preceding case, a modified Murphy procedure (split advancement of the tendo-Achilles to the medial and lateral calcaneus just posterior to the posterior subtalar joint) is my procedure of choice. As previously indicated, I prefer split transfer to complete transfer, especially in patients who have upper motor neuron disease. The lack of predictability in the firing of muscles with upper motor neuron disease can easily cause unanticipated iatrogenic deformity. With the more conventional Murphy procedure, the tendon is kept intact, placed centrally in the calcaneus from medial to lateral (frontal plane), and its position relative to the subtalar joint axis is, at best, an educated guess. The split tendon technique is a more pragmatic approach. An alternative technique is maintaining the tendon intact, including its distal flare, and creating a transverse trough in the calcaneus just posterior to the posterior facet. The broad insertion eliminates concern regarding its relationship to the subtalar joint axis. The split technique, however, has the added advantage of apportioning the split unequally to create increased muscle pull medially or laterally. When significant frontal plane malalignment exists, the split may be two thirds to one third rather than half and half. The larger tendinous portion is placed on the side favoring reduction of the frontal plane deformity.

Schoenhaus

Historically, the Murphy procedure has been employed for spastic equinus deformity; however, the procedure does not weaken the spastic muscle. It only shortens the lever arm. This patient needs a more aggressive approach, such as an open tendo-Achilles lengthening.

Harris

I am glad that this patient is 5 years old. Ankle equinus surgery is best done at this age or later because the recurrence rate is much lower. I would reassess the patient under general anesthesia. I suspect that there would be less apparent soleus "contracture." If this is my finding, then I would perform a gastrocnemius recession. If the contracture remains the same under anesthesia, then I would perform an open tendo-Achilles lengthening to gain maximal length. I would also assess the need for a limited posterior ankle release.

Question 6

What surgical follow-up would you employ?

Benard

Three weeks in a long-leg, non–weight-bearing cast with the foot in gravity equinus, followed by 3 weeks in a short-leg, neutral weight-bearing cast. I would prescribe gait training afterward, even in a 5-year-old.

Schoenhaus

A below-the-knee, non–weight-bearing cast in neutral position for 4 to 6 weeks and below-the-knee, partial weight-bearing casts for an additional 4 to 6 weeks. After the last cast, the patient would be placed in an AFO to be discontinued when the patient could ambulate as well with the AFO as without it. Then, active and passive dorsiflexion exercises would be started and physical therapy continued for 6 months. Night splints would be used to prevent contracture.

Harris

I would place the patient in non–weight-bearing casts with the ankle at neutral for at least 4 weeks. After that, I would apply walking casts with the ankle at neutral for an additional 2 weeks. At one of the cast changes, the patient would see the orthotist to begin fabrication of an AFO. After the patient is out of casts, he would return to physical therapy. The patient would wear the AFO at night also. Picking an end point to stop orthoses is case dependent. I have to confess that I continue the use of orthoses for a very long time. Perhaps, I should take the plunge and stop earlier, but I am excessively worried about recurrence.

Case 6—middle facet tarsal coalition

Chief complaint

A 12-year-old girl is referred because of a 6-week history of heel pain. She was seen at a screening program and referred because of her heel pain and bilateral flat feet.

Pertinent history

Initially, her pain was bilateral, but the left subsided. She was treated with ibuprofen and is now pain free for 2 weeks. The remainder of her past medical history is unremarkable.

Physical findings

The patient's gait is heel-toe on both sides, with both feet abducted to the line of progression equally. She is pronated in gait and stance. There is no limp. Table 6 shows biomechanical data. Bilateral anteroposterior, lateral, and Harris-Beath radiographs were obtained and are illustrated in Fig. 6A–D.

Question 1

What is your interpretation of these studies?

Table 6
Biomechanical data for case 6

Examination	Right	Left
Subtalar ROM inversion/eversion	10°/10°	10°/10°
Ankle ROM knee extended	+10°	+10°
Ankle ROM knee flexed	+12°	+12°
Tibial torsion	Out 25°	Out 20°
Popliteal angle	25°	25°
Hip ROM extended in/out	40°/30°	40°/30°
Hip ROM flexed in/out	40°/50°	40°/50°

Abbreviation: ROM, range of motion.

Benard

The clinical picture and biomechanical findings alone point strongly to tarsal coalition. Subtalar range of motion is significantly reduced. Anteroposterior and lateral radiographs demonstrate sclerotic changes in the region of the middle facet. The Harris-Beath views demonstrate complete absence of the middle facet, with an indication of an additional coalition of the posterior facet, although that

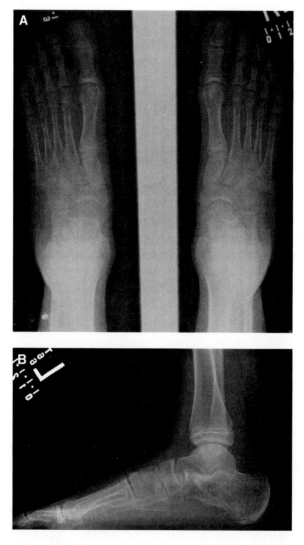

Fig. 6. Case 6—middle facet tarsal coalition. (*A*) Bilateral anteroposterior radiographs. (*B, C*) Lateral radiographs. (*D*) Harris-Beath radiographs. (*E*) Lateral MRI scan. (*F*) Coronal-plane MRI scan.

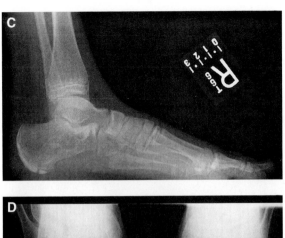

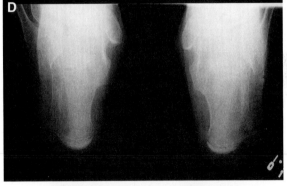

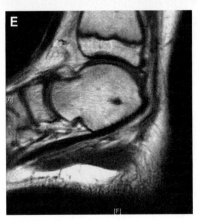

Fig. 6 (*continued*).

may be a radiographic artifact. I typically order Harris-Beath views at several different angles to appreciate a better picture of the subtalar joint. No clinical or historical findings are presented that would point to other etiologies. I also note that the patient's radiographic age is lagging her chronologic age, based on the appearance of her epiphyses.

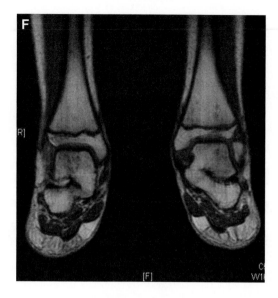

Fig. 6 (*continued*).

Schoenhaus

Both lateral radiographs show the classic "halo" sign with absence of the posterior subtalar facet. The right foot shows evidence of degenerative changes in the talonavicular joint with talonavicular beaking. The Harris-Beath views show absent posterior and middle facets.

Harris

The anteroposterior and lateral radiographs show very little in the area of pronation change. In fact, overall alignment would otherwise be acceptable. The lateral radiographs show some dorsal talonavicular remodeling. I would not label this arthrosis. The left lateral shows a halo sign, but this is less clear on the right. I do not see a middle facet on either lateral radiograph, and the posterior facets are not visualizing. The Harris-Beath projections show an abnormal sustentaculum tali on both sides. They slant inferomedially. I cannot see the middle facets at all. The posterior facets strike me as very narrow.

Question 2

MRI was obtained to further study this problem (see Fig. 6E, F). What is your interpretation of these studies?

Benard

Middle facet and possible partial posterior facet coalition, given the images presented. Although the diagnosis can be made with standard radiographs, MRI and CT studies are useful in determining the extent of the coalition. This information is valuable when surgical intervention is being considered.

Schoenhaus

The MRI findings suggest a complete osseous coalition of both posterior and middle facets.

Harris

The lateral MRI clearly shows the tendon of flexor hallucis longus passing under the sustentaculum tali. Because I cannot see a middle facet above the tendon, I would presume the presence of a synostotic coalition of the middle facet from this projection alone. The coronal-plane MRI shows complete bony coalition across both middle facets. The cuts show poorly developed posterior facets, but they are imaging pretty far anterior in these cuts. I would be cautious about interpreting the status of the posterior facets from either of these sets of images.

Question 3

Given the clinical history, what are your nonoperative recommendations?

Benard

The child's clinical symptoms are not severe. There is no peroneal "spasm" (a misnomer) present and I would not expect there to be, given the extent of the coalition. Although her relaxed calcaneal stance position is not given and no clinical photographs are presented, the radiographs do not indicate severe heel valgus or medial-lateral malalignment. Therefore, University of California Berkeley Laboratory Orthosis (UCBL-type) would be my choice, given the information presented.

Schoenhaus

Because the patient has an adequate range of motion at the ankle joint, accommodative orthoses should be fabricated. If the patient is still having pain after wearing these devices, then diagnostic talonavicular and peroneal injections could be attempted to help localize the site of her pain.

Harris

The fact that she is pain-free suggests that her symptoms are caused by maluse of motion segments outside of the subtalar joints. I would also start thinking about other possible causes of heel pain in this age group. Given the extent of the coalition, there cannot possibly be any motion there or in the posterior subtalar joint facets. I would look to the lateral ankle and the midtarsal joints as the site of the pain. I would design her orthoses to restrict coronal plane motion. I do not see her as a surgical problem at this time.

Question 4

Given the clinical history, what are your surgical recommendations?

Benard

I do not see this patient as a surgical candidate at this time. If orthotic therapy fails and her symptoms warrant surgical intervention in the future, then subtalar arthrodesis would be my choice. The extent of the coalition rules out simple resection of the medial aspect of the middle facet. In addition, although I perform fusions often enough in 12-year-olds, my criteria is the radiographic age rather than the chronologic age. The additional time gained with conservative care in this child would work to her advantage.

Schoenhaus

Unfortunately, given the involvement of the posterior facet, the surgical recommendation would be a triple arthrodesis.

Harris

If surgery were a last resort, there are several things I would not do. First, I believe that her coalitions are not resectable. Second, posterior facet fusion would probably not do much for this patient because the complex cannot move. Talonavicular fusion is indicated if that joint is the source of pain. Calcaneocuboid fusion remains controversial. Frequently, the pain is in the lateral ankle gutter because the calcaneus is fixed in eversion. The lateral side of the ankle is compressed. If this is the case, then a medial displacement osteotomy would center the calcaneus under the tibia and neutralize the cantilever effect of the lateral position of the calcaneus. Intelligent surgical intervention is dictated by the actual location of the pain. Keep in mind that the original complaint was heel pain, and it has resolved. Could this be calcaneal apophysitis in a child who also happens to have tarsal coalition?

Question 5

Given the clinical examination findings and the imaging data, how would you advise the family on prognosis?

Benard

In my experience, coalitions of this extent and at this location tend to create more significant symptoms later in life, which result from excessive stress on the adjacent joints. Although subtle, the child already demonstrates evidence of dorsal jamming at the right talonavicular joint. I would discuss the common clinical course of the condition, the need for orthotic control currently and long-term, and the possible need for surgery in the future.

Schoenhaus

Given the success with a course of anti-inflammatory medication, orthotic devices may be of benefit to reduce periarticular inflammation. The patient and family need to understand that arthritic changes are visible on radiographs, and that she will eventually need a fusion procedure. Use of orthoses would delay major fusion and spare the ankle and midtarsal joint arthrosis.

Harris

I see this as two separate issues. First, there is the resolved heel pain. Second, there is the issue of the extensive coalitions. I would tell the parents and the child that the heel pain may be unrelated to the coalitions, and I would suggest management for that diagnosis. The prognosis for apophysitis is guarded until closure of the apophyses. If pain in the heels recurs, then I would tell them that further work-up is indicated. The prognosis would depend on any subsequent diagnosis.

The issue of the coalition is more difficult. Some people go through their entire lives with these and never have any idea that they exist until they are incidentally discovered. Since the alignments of the feet are reasonable, orthoses may help stop the progression of the obvious remodeling changes that could lead to symptoms. If orthotic management fails, then she may require surgery. I would try to push this as far into the future as possible.

Case 7—tarsal coalition

Chief complaint

A 10-year-old boy has a 5-month history of foot pain and gait disturbance. Pain is continuous and rated as 5/10 on a visual analog scale. He indicates his medial and lateral calcaneal areas as the sites. He has tried nonsteroidal anti-inflammatory drugs, gel cushions, and shoe modifications without success.

Pertinent history

The child's history is unremarkable. His father is very disabled from bilateral middle facet tarsal coalitions. At age 42 years, the father is being considered as a candidate for triple arthrodesis.

Physical examination

The patient's gait has an apropulsive pattern but is otherwise heel-to-toe bilateral. The biomechanical data are shown in Table 7. Bilateral anteroposterior, lateral, and Harris-Beath radiographs were obtained and are illustrated in Fig. 7A–D.

Table 7
Biomechanical data for case 7

Examination	Right	Left
Subtalar ROM inversion/eversion	15°/7°	15°/7°
Ankle ROM knee extended	+7°	+7°
Ankle ROM knee flexed	+12°	+12°
Tibial torsion	Out 25°	Out 20°
Popliteal angle	25°	25°
Hip ROM extended in/out	25°/40°	25°/40°
Hip ROM flexed in/out	35°/45°	20°/45°

Abbreviation: ROM, range of motion.

Question 1

What is your interpretation of these studies?

Benard
Middle facet coalition, with secondary gastrocnemius equinus.

Schoenhaus
The Harris-Beath views are suspicious for middle facet coalitions because of the obliquity of the middle facet and the appearance of the posterior facet.

Harris
Overall alignment on the anteroposterior and lateral radiographs show acceptable static positioning. I cannot see a middle facet on either lateral radiograph. The Harris-Beath projections show obliquity of the sustentaculi and poor vision of the middle facets. I would diagnose middle facet coalitions from these studies.

Question 2

MRI was obtained to further study this problem (see Fig. 7E, F). What is your interpretation of these studies?

Benard
MRI findings support the diagnosis of middle facet coalition.

Schoenhaus
There are fibrous coalitions of the middle facets.

Harris
There are fibrous coalitions of the middle facets. The left shows more obliquity, but both are 100% involved.

Question 3

Given the clinical history, what are your nonoperative recommendations?

Benard
Maintain the child in UCBL-type orthoses until skeletally mature; re-evaluate with radiographs and MRI in the future.

Schoenhaus
Because the patient has an adequate range of motion at the ankle joint, accommodative orthoses would be fabricated. The patient would also be given a stretching regimen in an attempt to improve his hip internal rotation because this could contribute to pronatory heel pain. A diagnostic injection into the sinus tarsi would also be performed.

Harris
My initial treatment is similar to the last case. Orthotic management in an attempt to limit motion makes sense. UCBL orthoses would be my choice, and I would monitor the patient carefully.

Question 4

Given the clinical history, what are your surgical recommendations?

Benard
Based on the child's response to the orthoses, continue them to delay surgery until additional skeletal maturity is obtained or abandon them in favor of surgery. If the child proves to be recalcitrant to orthotic management, then I would evaluate the middle facet intraoperatively. If the clinical findings allow for resection of the medial aspect of the facet (which I doubt), then that would be my procedure of choice. If more extensive involvement is present, then I would perform extra-articular arthrodesis (modified Grice procedure) at this time. If the surgery can be delayed 2 to 3 years, based on updated imaging studies and clinical findings, then I would resect the middle facet (once again, not likely) or perform a standard subtalar arthrodesis.

Schoenhaus
My choice would be to resect 1 cm of the middle facets.

Harris
This is an interesting dilemma. I am still not sure how resection of the coalitions in these young children would hold up. Earlier "successes" tend to be-

come less rosy with time; however, there are no real adaptive changes, and they are fibrous coalitions. Resection would be a good choice of procedures. It has to be extensive and might result in excision of the entire sustentaculum tali. If the child and his parents understand the risks of failure and the subsequent need for additional surgery, then resection would be my choice of procedures.

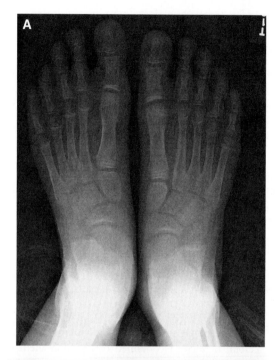

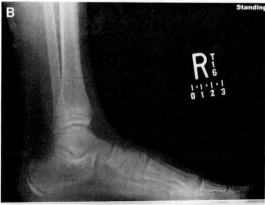

Fig. 7. Case 7—tarsal coalition. (*A*) Bilateral anteroposterior radiographs. (*B, C*) Lateral radiographs. (*D*) Harris-Beath radiographs. (*E, F*) MRI scans.

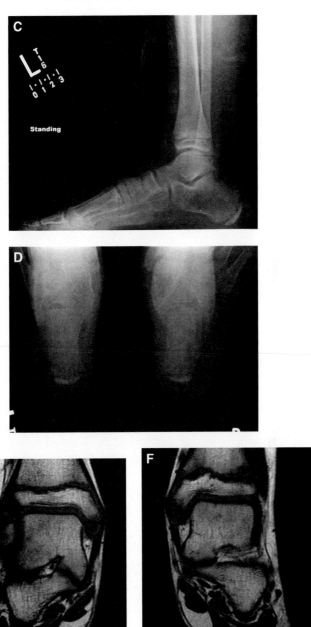

Fig. 7 (*continued*).

Question 5

Given the clinical examination findings and the imaging data, how would you advise the family on prognosis?

Benard

The child's father can corroborate the clinical course of the condition. I would discuss the likelihood of surgery in the short- or long-term because of the expected clinical course of partial middle facet coalition (chronic subtalar pain, secondary compensation and stress on surrounding joints, pedal malposition, decreased activity, and so forth).

Schoenhaus

Given the history of triple joint arthrosis in the patient's father, I would recommend resection of the middle facets. When the posterior facet is spared, resection of the middle facet can not only alleviate current symptomatology but, more important, also prevent future arthrosis of the talonavicular and calcaneocuboid joints.

Harris

This dilemma is the same as in the previous case. The father's history is not encouraging. The child may or may not follow the same course. Orthotic therapy may or may not achieve the anticipated goals. Only one thing is certain: as the patient matures, this condition will almost certainly become a synostotic coalition, and adaptive arthrosis is highly likely. The window for resection of the fibrous form of this coalition is rapidly closing. Although I have reservations about the long-term results of this procedure, I would recommend that they consider resection. I would also do extensive counseling about the procedure itself, the postoperative convalescence, the need for postoperative orthoses, and the guarded prognosis for success—all of which would be well documented.

ELSEVIER
SAUNDERS

Clin Podiatr Med Surg
23 (2006) 119–135

CLINICS IN
PODIATRIC
MEDICINE AND
SURGERY

The Ponseti Technique for Treatment of Talipes Equinovarus

Stephen Silvani, DPM

Orthopedic Department, The Permanente Medical Group and Kaiser Foundation Hospital at Walnut Creek, 1425 South Main Street, Walnut Creek, CA 94596, USA

The treatment of idiopathic talipes equinovarus (clubfoot) is historically challenging and usually consists of early manipulations followed by serial casting to maintain the correction [1–5]. This usually does not reduce the deformity completely and is followed by some surgical variation of extensive posterior-medial soft tissue release (Fig. 1A), biplanar pin fixation (see Fig. 1B), and more cast immobilization [2,3,6–8]. In relatively short-term follow-up (2–8 years) studies, 52% to 91% good or excellent results are reported. The results rapidly deteriorate, however, as seen in longer term follow-up reports (10–25 years after surgery) [9–11]. Surgical intervention for clubfoot has significant risks, complications, and the potential for a poorer prognosis as the patients age.

These feet are painful, stiff, scarred, weakened, and arthritic, and some have undergone multiple operations [1,12]. Complications caused by vascular embarrassment include wound slough, infections, ischemic necrosis, and limb loss [13–15]. Avascular necrosis of the talus, flat-top talus, and other rearfoot anatomic disruptions are seen after the soft tissue release (see Fig. 1C) [11,16]. Overcorrection with heel valgus, pes plano valgus, and calcaneus deformity as well as loss of surgical correction with residual equinus, heel varus, and forefoot adductus is commonly seen [8,17,18]. Limb length discrepancies have been reported after releases for unilateral deformities [19].

In 1950, at the University of Iowa, Ignacio Ponseti perfected his method of manipulation and casting of idiopathic clubfoot after thoroughly elucidating the kinematics and pathologic anatomy of the deformity. This simple technique avoided the complete invasive soft tissue release surgery and produced a functional, supple, and plantigrade foot. These feet are normal looking, pain-free, and without calluses and do not require modified shoes. His satisfactory results

E-mail address: Stephen.silvani@kp.org

0891-8422/06/$ – see front matter © 2006 Elsevier Inc. All rights reserved.
doi:10.1016/j.cpm.2005.10.002   *podiatric.theclinics.com*

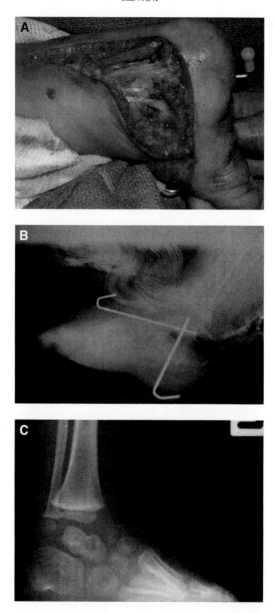

Fig. 1. (*A*) The extensive dissection necessary for a posterior medial clubfoot release is seen through this Turco approach. (*B*) An intraoperative radiograph shows the gaping hard-to-close Cincinnati approach and the pin immobilization of the subtalar and talonavicular joints. (*C*) A typical postoperative result is seen here. Note the posterior rotation of the fibula on this lateral view, the distorted flat-top talus, and the navicular riding dorsally on the talus.

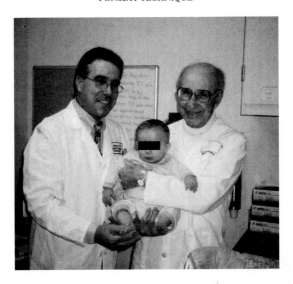

Fig. 2. The author and Dr. Ignacio Ponseti (*left*) hold an infant with a well-corrected right clubfoot.

were first reported in 1963 [20], and a later review of patients 25 to 42 years after treatment revealed a high percentage of optimum results [21]. His life's work, passion, and research as well as fundamentals of his manipulation were chronicled in his book, *Congenital Clubfoot*, in 1996 [22].

I was fortunate to have been trained by Dr. Ponseti when he visited my facility several times for in-service sessions and follow-up of his West Coast patients (Fig. 2). It was inspiring to see the admiration on the parent's faces and the well-corrected functional feet of the children when they met with this guru. I have been using his technique on idiopathic as well as some syndromic clubfoot since early 2000. A review of the first 57 clubfeet treated by this method at our facility revealed that 95% were corrected without a posterior medial release [23]. Many of these infants had previously been scheduled for the full surgical release and were spared the intervention.

This article outlines the manipulation, casting, and percutaneous Achilles tenotomy; provides technique pearls; and reviews the outcomes of this efficacious method of treating clubfoot.

Pathoanatomy and technique of manipulation

The pathoanatomy of the clubfoot must be thoroughly understood before the manipulation and reduction make sense. The talus is locked in equinus in the ankle mortise by the tight Achilles tendon. The tarsal bones distal to the talus (calcaneus, cuboid, and navicular) are adducted and inverted. The forefoot has a cavus position as a result of pronation on the rearfoot, mainly because of plantarflexion of the first metatarsal.

To reduce this anatomy, the tarsal bones must be abducted with the foot in supination and all three rearfoot joints remodeled congruently. The supinated forefoot remains parallel to the inverted rearfoot. Dorsal pressure on the first ray reduces the cavus, which is caused by plantarflexion of the first metatarsal. At first, this seems counterintuitive, because the foot is supinated in relation to the leg. Simultaneously, the navicular glides plantarly and laterally in front of the head of the talus, the cuboid slides and moves in front of the calcaneus, and the calcaneus rolls laterally out from underneath the talus (Fig. 3). The foot is simultaneously abducted at the subtalar joint, Chopart's joint, the navicular cuneiform joint, and Lisfranc's joint without any pronation of the foot. It is only after the calcaneus abducts from under the talus (opening up the talocalcaneal angle) that it can be dorsiflexed by the Achilles tenotomy. The calcaneus is ready to be dorsiflexed when the foot is abducted approximately 70° externally. The reduction is gradual, with stretching of the tarsal ligaments, and is maintained by casting. The foot is "massaged" into the corrected position without undue force or bone and cartilage damage.

Another basic tenet of this technique is never touching the calcaneus during manipulation. Ponseti referred to this as Kite's error, because Kite [1] advocated counterpressure at the calcaneocuboid joint level while manipulating the forefoot. Holding or lateral pressure on the calcaneus prevents its abduction and its rolling out from underneath the talus to reduce the heel varus and, later, the equinus. Firm pressure on the lateral head of the talus keeps it stable in the ankle mortise while the foot distally is abducted out from underneath it (Fig. 4). This lateral

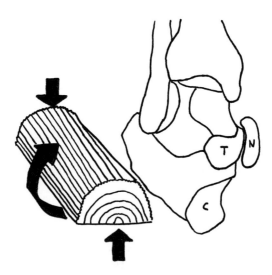

Fig. 3. The anterior portion of the calcaneus in the clubfoot lies beneath the head of the talus, causing the varus and equinus of the heel. This is similar to a log floating in water. The anterior end cannot elevate until it is rolled out from underneath the talus. This abduction reduces the heel varus and allows the Achilles tenotomy to reduce the equinus.

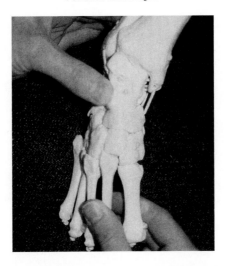

Fig. 4. The forefoot is supinated and abducted while counterpressure is applied to the talar head. The calcaneus is never touched during the manipulation.

talar head pressure prevents the external rotation of the fibula on the tibia, an iatrogenic deformity so commonly seen in feet treated traditionally.

One must palpate the relation of the navicular tuberosity to the medial malleolus. The shorter this distance, the more severe is the clubfoot. Monitoring this interval documents progress in swinging the foot into abduction. When abducting the forefoot, the ease of moving the navicular away from the malleolus also correlates with the severity of the deformity.

Classification

There are many degrees of severity and rigidity found in idiopathic clubfoot. Three main classification systems are commonly used to assess these feet. The modified Dimeglio-Bensahel method uses eight components for a total of 20 points [24]. The higher the score, the more severe is the foot. The Catterall-Pirani system consists of six features, with a higher score indicating a more rigid foot [25,26]. The Hospital for Joint Diseases Functional Rating scheme rates six components for a best score of 60 points [27,28]. With proper replication of the Ponseti technique and documentation with these functional rating systems, ongoing studies can follow corrected children as they mature and provide a database for future study. More studies are now being reported that are replicating and independently confirming the high success rate that Ponseti has claimed all along [11,21,23]. These classification schemes ensure that similar deformities are being compared.

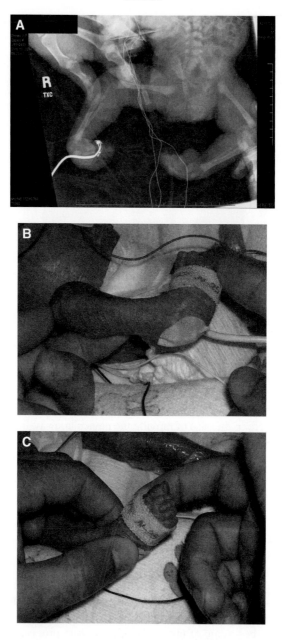

Fig. 5. (*A*) A premature neonate with an unknown myopathy presents with severely rigid bilateral clubfeet and a left congenital dislocated hip. (*B*) The rigid clubfoot as it appears before manipulation. (*C*) Early reduction is seen after brief manipulation, and good correction was achieved after several casts.

Ponseti does not use a severity classification scheme because he states that the degree of deformity is not necessarily related to the ease of correction [29]. I have personally treated several neonates with a high Dimeglio score who responded early and completely to manipulation and tenotomy.

The Ponseti technique was developed for and works best on nonsyndromic idiopathic clubfoot. When applying this technique to infants with underlying neuromuscular disease or arthrogryposis (Fig. 5), I have found its success to be slightly less than of the idiopathic clubfoot. Some of these more challenging feet require the traditional posterior medial release after failing the Ponseti technique.

Treatment protocol

The typical number of manipulation and cast sessions held until correction or tenotomy is three to seven, with four to five being average. Infants greater than 6 months old and those having prior treatment usually take longer for correction. There is no documented reason to take an older infant to surgery before trying the properly performed Ponseti technique [29]. Ideally, the visits are from 5 to 7 days apart.

Infants are treated as soon as possible after birth, although this method has been shown to work on babies as old as 6 months to 2 years of age and in patients who had previous failed manipulations [29]. I have started casting neonates in our postpartum rooms as soon as the vernix was washed away. Usually, we wait until the day the baby is discharged, when we manipulate and apply the first cast (Fig. 6).

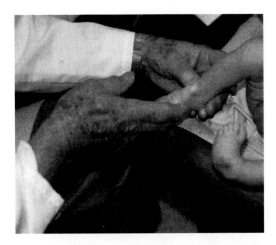

Fig. 6. The proper hand position is demonstrated, and counterpressure is only applied to the lateral talar head.

Thin cast padding (Webril; Kendall Company, Mansfield, Massachusetts) is used by only overlapping half of the roll width so as to prevent cast slippage with loss of correction (Fig. 7). A short ring cut from a cast stocking roll used proximally and folded over the plaster prevents groin irritation. Although Ponseti removes the cast with a cast knife blade, I have had minimal problems with orthopedic technicians using a cast saw, even with the thin padding. A medial and lateral strip of 1-in wide foam tape placed over the padding where the cast saw cuts prevents saw burns. The only acceptable casting material is plaster, especially extra–fast-setting types (Gypsona; Smith and Nephew, Germantown, Wisconsin), because of its molding ability. Hot water is necessary for faster setting times, whereas continued manipulation is performed until the cast is fully hardened. A toe-to-groin cast is necessary to prevent the talus from rotating in the ankle. The correction gained by the manipulation would be lost if a short leg cast were applied.

The first manipulation concentrates on supinating the forefoot to reduce the cavus component by gently dorsiflexing the first metatarsal head. This is a key step in this technique [30,31]; if it is not performed, the result is a stiff non-reducible foot. The next several manipulations and casts laterally mobilize the calcacaneopedal block over the talar head fulcrum until the foot is abducted approximately 70° (Fig. 8). This usually occurs after three to four weekly visits. If the Achilles tenotomy is attempted before the foot is fully externally rotated and the anterior part of the calcaneus is rotated from underneath the talus, incomplete reduction of the equinus occurs.

If the foot does not have at least 10° to 15° of dorsiflexion, a complete percutaneous Achilles tenotomy is necessary. One last cast is placed for 3 weeks

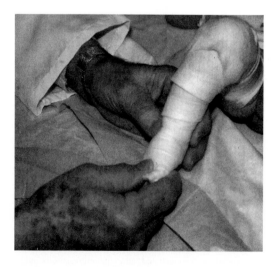

Fig. 7. Thin cast padding is used to allow the cast to hold the correction without slipping.

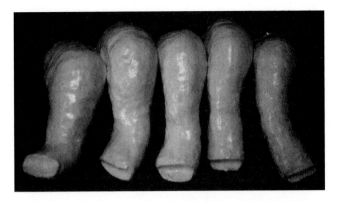

Fig. 8. The first cast is the supinated one shown on the right, and the reduction of the deformity can be seen. The last cast after the tenotomy with good ankle dorsiflexion is shown on the left.

before using the abduction bar. In marginal cases, I have found that it is better to err on the side of doing the tenotomy than not. Retracting fibrosis continues to develop, and further equinus can occur in feet that seemed acceptable at the end of casting. It was then necessary to remanipulate, recast, and perform the tenotomy anyway. A recent study of 50 clubfeet demonstrated a 72% tenotomy rate and predictive values of more severe Pirani and Demeglio scores, indicating the need for the tenotomy [32]. Another retrospective review showed a 91% tenotomy rate when less than 10° of dorsiflexion was achieved after casting the foot to 70° of abduction [33].

The Achilles tenotomy can easily be performed as an office procedure under local anesthesia. There is no need for the risk and expense of general anesthesia

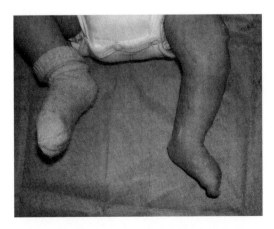

Fig. 9. The foot is now fully abducted and ready for the tenotomy. Some cast saw irritation is seen as well as the occlusive film holding on the application of EMLA topical anesthetic cream.

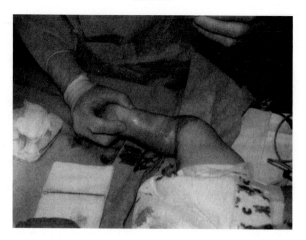

Fig. 10. An assistant firmly holds the leg after the sterile preparation.

and a trip to the operating room. A topical local anesthetic cream (EMLA, Astra Zeneca, Wilmington, Delaware) placed under an occlusive dressing for 30 to 45 minutes provides enough numbness for the procedure (Fig. 9). An assistant holds the foot securely dorsiflexed while the foot and leg are prepared and covered by an aperture drape (Fig. 10). With the parents out of the treatment room, a blade (long cataract or 67 Beaver blade; Becton Dickinson and Company, Franklin Lakes, New Jersey) is introduced from a medial direction, just anterior and parallel to the Achilles tendon (Fig. 11). It is then rotated posteriorly and transects the tendon with an audible and palpable pop. A defect should be felt in

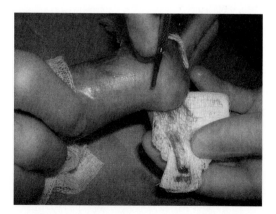

Fig. 11. The blade is introduced from the medial side and then rotated posteriorly to tenotomize the Achilles tendon. The tip is kept away from the neurovascular bundles.

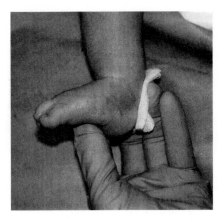

Fig. 12. A pressure bandage is applied to stop the bleeding before the final dressing and cast are applied.

the tendon, and the infant should not be able to forcibly plantarflex when kicking. A pressure gauze dressing is applied (Fig. 12), and 1% lidocaine (2–3 mL) is infiltrated around the tendon (Fig. 13). This is not done before the tenotomy, because the wheal and/or volume of local anesthetic obscures the tendon borders, making it impossible to palpate, and jeopardizes blade placement. No suture is necessary, and a fresh sterile gauze dressing is placed under the last maximally dorsiflexed and abducted cast, which stays on for 3 weeks.

Using this technique, one has control of the blade tip and can avoid the major vascular structures. Some venous bleeding is encountered, which is easily

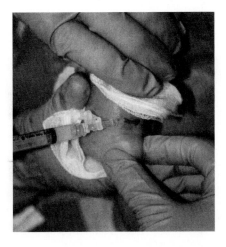

Fig. 13. The local anesthetic is injected after the tenotomy is performed so that the tendon remains palpable.

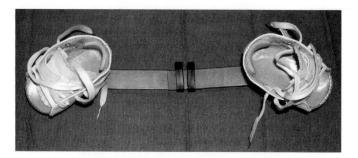

Fig. 14. The shoes are externally rotated 70° on the bar for bilateral clubfeet.

stopped by brief pressure. Few incidents of major vessel damage are reported. Nevertheless, 4 of 200 Achilles tenotomies in one review had major bleeding complications, probably because of peroneal artery and saphenous vein damage [33]. If Doppler studies are inconclusive, the authors recommended an arteriogram to document vascular anatomy, which can be aberrant in congenital deformities. Others recommend using a large-bore needle to saw through the tendon, thus avoiding the use of a blade [34]. The tendon is fully regenerated when the cast is removed in 3 weeks as a result of the incredible healing properties of infants.

The straight last shoe size is measured before the tenotomy, and the shoes and bar are ordered at that time. After the last cast removal, the feet are placed in the shoe fitted with a Denis Browne–type adjustable bar. The length of the bar is equal to the width of the patient's shoulders. For the clubfoot side, the shoe is abducted 70°; the normal side is abducted 45° (Fig. 14). An upward bend of 15° in the middle of the bar maintains the equinus correction (Fig. 15). The infant

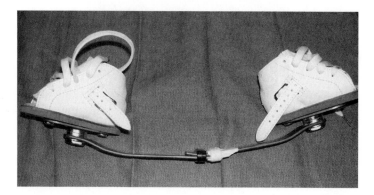

Fig. 15. The bar is bent 15° upward to keep the feet in dorsiflexion and prevent reoccurrence of the equinus.

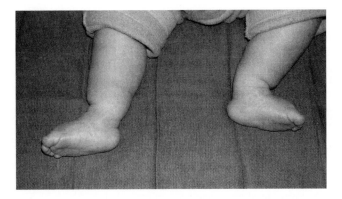

Fig. 16. The typical appearance of well-corrected bilateral clubfeet 3 months after the tenotomy is shown.

remains in the shoe-bar combination 24 hours a day 7 days a week for 3 to 4 months and then all night and during nap times for 3 to 4 years to prevent relapses (Fig. 16).

There is a short learning curve for parents to place the feet into the shoes properly, making sure that the heel is all the way down and then tightening the laces on a squirming infant. Shoe stretcher devices can enlarge a posterior heel bulge, and padding can be added around the shoe counter to prevent the heel from slipping up and returning to equinus (Fig. 17). Some parents wrap the bar with pipe foam insulation or tape to prevent the bar from causing injuries to others or to the bed sheets when the infant learns to kick with both legs.

Lack of compliance in properly using the bar directly leads to relapses and the need for further treatment by 17 times the rate in compliant parents [29]. Ponseti

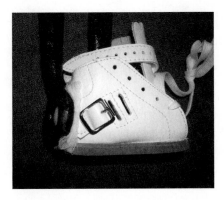

Fig. 17. The heel is firmly held by the posterior bulge created by shoe stretching.

defined a relapse as any return of the cavus, adductus, varus, or equinus. Initially, patients are treated by repeat manipulations and casting and, if necessary, another tenotomy. In the older child, if the anterior tibialis tendon strongly supinates the foot, its transfer to the third cuneiform can correct the deformity.

Discussion

The literature is now replete with independently performed peer-reviewed studies confirming the excellent efficacy of a properly performed Ponseti technique, managing the clubfoot deformity without the need for extensive surgical intervention in greater than 95% of cases [11,21,23,28,31,32]. Although perfect anatomic or radiographic correction is not achieved, a functional foot is created that lasts for decades (Fig. 18) [21].

Imaging modalities have now shown unequivocally the anatomic restoration of more normal anatomy and less pathologic residuals with the Ponseti method as compared with traditional techniques. Assessment of the relation of the tarsal bones before and after Ponseti treatment by plain radiographs is difficult because

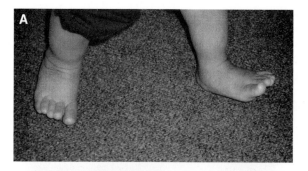

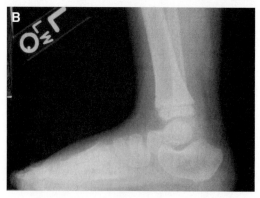

Fig. 18. A satisfactory result is seen clinically (*A*) and radiographically (*B*) in this 4-year-old child after Ponseti treatment.

of the radiographically silent navicular in infants; yet, the reduction of the adductus and equinus is seen. Using MRI, it has been shown that not only is there correction of the abnormal alignment of the tarsal bones but that actual changes in the abnormal shapes of the tarsal osteochondral angles occur through this manipulation [35]. Similarly, real-time ultrasound has demonstrated dynamically the movement of the bones toward their reduced position during the manipulations as well as the maintenance of the correction [36].

The main factor leading to relapse was failure to use the shoes attached to the bar in external rotation for the proper length of time [28,30,37]. No correlation was found between the severity of the deformity, age at initiation of treatment, previous treatment, parental marital status, or income level and reoccurrence. Only parental educational status (high school or less) was a risk factor for relapse. The use of the bar and shoes for the proper length of time is mandatory, and its importance must be stressed to the parents. Late recurrence (at 8 years of age) is extremely rare but can occur, and the parents must be aware of this possibility [38].

Traditionally, parents have sought information on medical problems from health care providers. Today, the Internet is a major source of information for patients and has been credited with disseminating and popularizing the Ponseti technique among parents and physicians alike. Parents of children with clubfoot share experiences and opinions in support group chat rooms and seek information on Ponseti's web page, which is posted on the Virtual Hospital at the University of Iowa [39]. We have parents present who are "doctor shopping" for a physician using this technique after having a clubfoot visualized on screening intrauterine ultrasound (Fig 19).

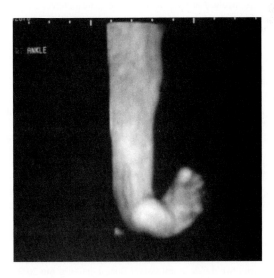

Fig. 19. An expectant mother presented with this intrauterine ultrasound of a fetus with clubfoot when looking for a physician who performed the Ponseti technique.

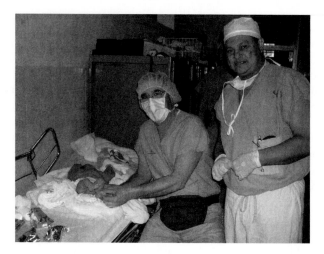

Fig. 20. The author demonstrates the manipulation of a clubfoot while on a medical trip to Hondouras.

In conclusion, the Ponseti method of clubfoot management is quite effective in producing functional outcomes. It limits the need for extensive surgery, is reproducible and easy to learn, and is rapidly becoming the standard all over the world for the treatment of talipes equinovarus (Fig. 20).

References

[1] Kite JH. Principles involved in the treatment of congenital clubfoot. J Bone Joint Surg [Am] 1939;21:595–606.

[2] McKay DW. New concepts of and approach to clubfoot treatment: section II: correction of the clubfoot. J Pediatr Orthop 1983;3:10–21.

[3] Nather A, Bose K. Conservative and surgical management of the clubfoot. J Pediatr Orthop 1987;7:42–8.

[4] Zimbler S. Nonoperative management of the equinovarus foot: long term results. In: Simons GW, editor. The clubfoot. New York: Springer-Verlag; 1994. p. 191–3.

[5] Cummins RJ, Lovell WW. Operative treatment on congenital idiopathic clubfoot. J Bone Joint Surg Am 1988;70:1108–12.

[6] Carroll NC. Clubfoot: what have we learned in the last quarter century? J Pediatr Orthop 1997; 17:1–2.

[7] Carroll NC, Gross RH. Operative management of clubfoot. Orthopedics 1990;13:1285–96.

[8] Turco VJ. Resistant congenital clubfoot: one-stage posteromedial release with internal fixation: a follow-up report of a fifteen-year experience. J Bone Joint Surg Am 1979;61:805–14.

[9] Green AD, Lloyd-Roberts GC. The results of early posterior release in resistant clubfeet: a long term review. J Bone Joint Surg Br 1985;67:588–93.

[10] Hutchins PM, Foster BK, Paterson DC, et al. Long term results of early surgical release in clubfeet. J Bone Joint Surg Br 1985;67:791–9.

[11] Ippolito E, Farsetti P, Caterini R, et al. Long-term comparative results in patients with congenital clubfoot treated with two different protocols. J Bone Joint Surg Am 2003;85:1286–94.

[12] Aronson J, Puskarich CL. Deformity and disability from treated clubfoot. J Pediatr Orthop 1990; 10:109–19.

[13] Dobbs MB, Gordon JE, Schoenecker PL. Absent posterior tibial artery associated with idiopathic clubfoot. J Bone Joint Surg Am 2004;86:599–602.

[14] Hootnick DR, Packard DS, Levinsohn EM, et al. Ischemic necrosis following clubfoot surgery: the purple hallux sign. J Pediatr Orthop 2004;13:315–22.

[15] Hootnick DR, Packard DS, Levinsohn EM. Necrosis leading to amputation following clubfoot surgery. Foot Ankle 1990;10:312–6.

[16] Cummins RJ, Bashore CJ, Bookout CB, et al. Avascular necrosis of the talus after McKay clubfoot release for idiopathic congenital clubfoot. J Pediatr Orthop 2001;21:221–4.

[17] Weseley MS, Barenfeld PA, Barrett N. Complications of the treatment of clubfoot. Clin Orthop 1972;84:93–6.

[18] McKay DW. New concept of and approach to clubfoot treatment: section III—evaluation and results. J Pediatr Orthop 1983;3:141–8.

[19] Noonan KJ, Meyers AM, Kayes K. Leg length discrepancy in unilateral congenital clubfoot following surgical treatment. Iowa Orthop J 2001;24:60–4.

[20] Ponseti IV, Smoley EN. Congenital clubfoot: the results of treatment. J Bone Joint Surg Am 1963;45:261–75.

[21] Cooper DM, Dietz FR. Treatment of idiopathic clubfoot. A thirty year follow-up. J Bone Joint Surg Am 1995;77:1477–89.

[22] Ponseti IV. Congenital clubfoot. Fundamentals of treatment. New York: Oxford University Press; 1996.

[23] Colburn MW, Williams M. Evaluation of the treatment of idiopathic clubfoot by using the Ponseti method. J Foot Ankle Surg 2003;42:259–67.

[24] Dimeglio A, Bensahel H, Souchet P, et al. Classification of clubfoot. J Pediatr Orthop B 1995;4:129–36.

[25] Catterall A. A method of assessment of the clubfoot. Clin Orthop 1991;264:48–53.

[26] Pirani S. A method of assessing the virgin clubfoot. Presented at the Pediatric Orthopedic Society of North America. Orlando, February 16–21, 1995.

[27] Atar D, Lehman WB, Grant AD, et al. Revision surgery in clubfeet. Clin Orthop 1992;283: 223–30.

[28] Lehman WB, Mohaideen A, Madan S, et al. A method for the early evaluation of the Ponseti (Iowa) technique for the treatment of idiopathic clubfoot. J Pediatr Orthop B 2003;12:133–40.

[29] Morcuende JA, Dolan LA, Dietz FR, et al. Radical reduction in the rate of extensive corrective surgery for clubfoot using the Ponseti method. An Pediatr (Barc) 2004;113:376–80.

[30] Ponseti IV. Comon errors in the treatment of congenital clubfoot. Int Orthop 1997;21:137–41.

[31] Frick SL. The Ponseti method of treatment for congenital clubfoot: importance of maximal supination in initial casting. Orthopedics 2005;18:63–5.

[32] Scher DM, Feldman DS, Van Bosse HJP, et al. Predicting the need for tenotomy in the Ponseti method for correction of clubfeet. J Pediatr Orthop 2004;24:349–52.

[33] Dobbs MB, Gordon JE, Walton T, et al. Bleeding complications following percutaneous tendo-Achilles tenotomy in the treatment of clubfoot deformity. J Pediatr Orthop 2004;24:353–7.

[34] Minkowitz B, Finkelstein BI, Bleicher M. Percutaneous tendo-Achilles lengthening with a large gauge needle: a modification of the Ponseti technique for correction of idiopathic clubfoot. J Foot Ankle Surg 2004;43:263–5.

[35] Pirani S, Zeznik L, Hodges D. Magnetic resonance imaging study of the congenital clubfoot treated with the Ponseti method. J Pediatr Orthop 2001;21:719–26.

[36] Kuhns LR, Koujok K, Hall JM, et al. Ultrasound of the navicular during the simulated Ponseti maneuver. J Pediatr Orthop 2003;23:243–5.

[37] Dobbs MB, Rudzki JR, Purcell DB, et al. Factors predictive of outcome after use of the Ponseti method for the treatment of idiopathic clubfeet. J Bone Joint Surg Am 2004;86:22–7.

[38] Dobbs MB, Corley CL, Morcuende JA, et al. Late recurrence of clubfoot deformity: a 45-year followup. Clin Orthop 2003;411:188–92.

[39] Morcuende JA, Egbert M, Ponseti IV. The effect of the Internet in the treatment of congenital idiopathic clubfoot. Iowa Orthop J 2003;23:83–6.

ELSEVIER
SAUNDERS

Clin Podiatr Med Surg
23 (2006) 137–166

CLINICS IN
PODIATRIC
MEDICINE AND
SURGERY

External Fixation for the Foot and Ankle in Children

Bradley M. Lamm, DPM*, Shawn C. Standard, MD,
Ian J. Galley, MD[1], John E. Herzenberg, MD, Dror Paley, MD

*Rubin Institute for Advanced Orthopedics, Sinai Hospital of Baltimore, 2401 West Belvedere Avenue,
Baltimore, MD 21215, USA*

This article provides an overview and an update about the evolving indications and applications of external fixation for the pediatric foot and ankle. During the last decade, there have been many advances in technology and preoperative deformity planning for external fixation. The principles of deformity correction have evolved as an essential component for successful application of external fixation. Improved technology, such as the Taylor spatial frame and hydroxy-apatite-coated external fixator pins, has expanded the indications and applications of external fixation for pediatric foot and ankle conditions.

External fixation can be used for gradual osseous and soft tissue deformity correction or to stabilize an acute correction. During external fixation treatment, doctors have access to soft tissues for wound care. External fixation allows for fine-tuning of residual deformity correction during the postoperative period and can allow for joint range of motion and early weight bearing. Theoretically, these advantages should lessen disuse osteoporosis and maintain joint range of motion and cartilage nutrition; however, despite the use of "walking rings" (Fig. 1), disuse osteopenia of the foot bones remains a problem in children (Fig. 2).

One disadvantage of external fixation is the specialized surgical expertise that is required for construction and postoperative management. Complications such as pin-site infections are common; however, most complications are minor

* Corresponding author.

E-mail address: blamm@lifebridgehealth.org (B.M. Lamm).

[1] P.O. Box 3092, Melbourne Street, North Adelaide, Adelaide, South Australia, Australia. Address after December 2005: Tauranga Hospital, 257 Oropi Gorge Road, Pyes Pa, RD3, Tauranga, New Zealand.

0891-8422/06/$ – see front matter © 2006 Elsevier Inc. All rights reserved.
doi:10.1016/j.cpm.2005.10.007   *podiatric.theclinics.com*

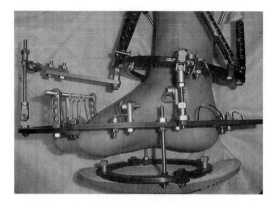

Fig. 1. Walking ring permits the patient to bear weight during the treatment.

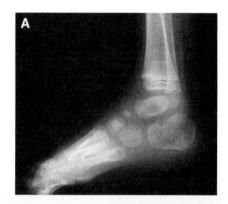

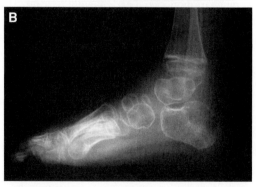

Fig. 2. Disuse osteopenia can occur with extended treatment periods. (*A*) Preoperative lateral view radiograph of the foot and ankle shows normal bone density. (*B*) Generalized pedal osteopenia is observed in the lateral view radiograph after external fixation is removed. Thus, weight bearing is encouraged with a walking ring.

and can be addressed nonoperatively. Typically, when operative intervention is required, treatment can continue while the complication is being addressed [1,2].

Historical perspective

External fixation and limb lengthening have been used for more than a century. Codivilla [3] has been credited as being the first physician to perform and report on limb lengthening, in 1904. A variety of heavy and awkward external fixator devices that often confined a patient to bed were used together with bone regeneration in the first half of the twentieth century. Professor Gavril Abramovich Ilizarov, working in Kurgan during the 1950s, developed a portable, modular, circular fixator with transosseous tensioned wire fixation. He relied on bone regeneration in the distraction gap and recommended a minimally invasive osteotomy. Ilizarov applied his techniques to the treatment of deformity, limb-length discrepancy, nonunion, osteomyelitis, fractures, and bone defects. He worked in relative obscurity until 1967, when he treated an infected nonunion sustained by Valery Brumel, an Olympic high jump champion. Ilizarov was invited to Italy in 1981, and his method was introduced to Europe by Italian orthopedic surgeons from Lecco, Bergamo, and Milan. The Ilizarov method was introduced to North America by Dr. Dror Paley in 1986 after he spent 6 months studying in Italy and the Soviet Union [4].

Although the Ilizarov method remained unknown to the English-speaking world until the mid-1980s, one of the first English language publications about Ilizarov, Kurgan, and the Ilizarov method was published in the *Journal of the American Podiatry Association* in 1973 (currently called the *Journal of the American Podiatric Medical Association*) [5]. It was not until 1996 that another article about Ilizarov's technique was published in the podiatric literature [6]. Today, the Ilizarov technique is widely used by a growing number of orthopedic and podiatric surgeons.

New technology

In 1994, Dr. J. Charles Taylor and his brother, engineer Harold Taylor, developed the Taylor spatial frame (Smith & Nephew, Memphis, Tennessee) [7]. The Taylor spatial frame, which modified the Ilizarov apparatus, is a circular external fixator that uses a Stewart platform and projective geometry by way of a computer program to allow for precise gradual deformity correction in any plane. New hardware and software have been developed specifically for the foot and ankle. Improvements in spatial frame technology have increased the potential applications for complex deformity correction of the foot and ankle. The Internet-based Total Residual computer software program (www.spatialframe.com; Smith & Nephew) has been substantially modified to make it more specific for foot and ankle correction.

Soft tissue contracture

Contractures of the soft tissue structures around the foot can result from a multitude of causes, including previous trauma, surgery, compartment syndromes, congenital abnormalities, burns, radiation, and a variety of neurologic conditions [8]. The contractures range from simple equinus contractures of the ankle to complex multiplanar deformities of the foot and ankle with associated skeletal malalignment and joint degeneration [9]. It is important to identify bony deformity that can mimic soft tissue contractures. For example, distal tibial procurvatum, forefoot equinus, and flattop talus can mimic an ankle equinus contracture [7]. It is also important to recognize that osseous deformities can coexist or contribute to soft tissue contractures.

Skeletal malalignment and soft tissue contractures can be treated simultaneously with external fixation, although the constructs can become very complex. The causes of soft tissue contractures can be further divided into extra-articular, intra-articular, or extra- and intra-articular causes. The extra-articular causes of ankle contractures might involve muscles such as the gastrocnemius, soleus, tibialis posterior, flexor digitorum longus, and flexor hallucis longus muscles. Intra-articular causes include capsular contractures, joint adhesions, and joint mice. In addition, joint incongruity can be present. Small corrections, such as $10°$ of ankle equinus, can be achieved with traditional soft tissue releases and tendon lengthening [7,10].

Large acute corrections might require soft tissue expanders [11], extensive soft tissue release, shortening osteotomy, or microvascular free-tissue transfer [12] to address soft tissue coverage. A safer alternative is gradual correction with an external fixator [1,2,13,14], which reduces the morbidity of large corrections, especially in the presence of abnormal soft tissues such as scars, burns, and unstable skin. External fixation allows for gradual distraction of abnormal soft tissues without extensive open exposures through them. The correction can be achieved purely through soft tissue distraction, or it can be combined with limited soft tissue releases. Avoiding tendon releases lessens the chance of over-lengthening or excessively weakening the muscle-tendon unit. Gradual correction of the foot and ankle is also less likely to compromise the nerves and the vascular supply. The risk can be further reduced by decompressing the posterior tibial neurovascular bundle at the time of frame application. The authors often perform tarsal tunnel release before correcting an equinus contracture that is more than $10°$ to $20°$, especially in the presence of associated varus. Such releases can also be performed on an as-needed basis during the course of gradual correction. If any neurologic compromise occurs during gradual distraction, the rate of distraction can be slowed or temporarily stopped to allow for recovery. Nerve decompression should be considered when the nerve function does not improve or when any new motor deficit is noted. Contractures should be overcorrected and held with the fixator for a minimum of 4 to 6 weeks to allow for soft tissue adaptation. To prevent recurrence, the position should be maintained with a cast for approximately 4 weeks and with functional bracing thereafter. Any motor imbalance should be addressed by subsequent tendon transfer or bracing to prevent recurrence.

External fixators that are used to correct equinus contractures can be constructed as uniaxial hinge (constrained) or no hinge (unconstrained). The Taylor spatial frame correction is performed by means of a virtual hinge (Fig. 3). The constrained fixator has a single hinge centered on the center of rotation of the joint being treated. It is typically applied to large hinge joints, such as the elbow, knee, or ankle, that comprise a single and easily defined axis of rotation and correction. The constrained fixator allows for range of motion of the joint during contracture correction. An ankle fixator should be constructed to allow for distraction of the ankle joint space during the deformity correction, and fixation should be applied to the talus and the calcaneus to prevent overdistraction of the subtalar joint. Unconstrained constructs are used for multiaxial, multijoint corrections (eg, clubfoot) [7].

Idiopathic clubfoot

Occasionally, Ilizarov techniques are indicated for older infants who have primary clubfoot deformities and experience a delay in diagnosis. The primary indication in the authors' practice, however, is for toddlers and children who have recurrent clubfoot deformities and have previously undergone extensive open surgery and for selected older children and adults who have residual clubfoot deformities. The treatment of these complex deformities in young children is performed with multiplanar external fixators (eg, Ilizarov) in an unconstrained fashion [13,15–18]. Children younger than 8 years can be treated by soft tissue and joint distraction, whereas children 8 years and older are typically treated with distraction osteotomies. Younger children are treated with soft tissue and joint distraction because they still possess some degree of biologic plasticity (remodeling potential) of their bones and cartilage (Fig. 4).

The Ilizarov method of joint and soft tissue distraction is analogous to treating infants with serial casting. With casting, pressure is applied to the skin, and the joints primarily experience compressive forces. In contrast, the Ilizarov method applies distraction forces across the joints. The tight soft tissues are stretched rather than surgically released, avoiding extensive intra-articular fibrosis and pericapsular scarring. Treating a patient with tendon lengthening can alter the Blix curve of the musculotendinous unit and cause permanent weakness. The risk is largely avoided with distraction.

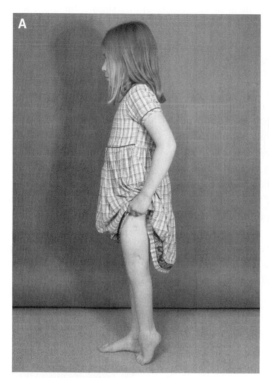

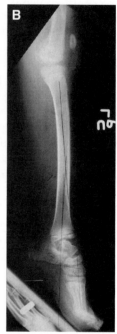

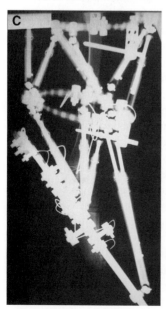

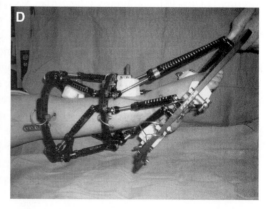

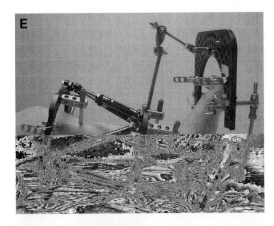

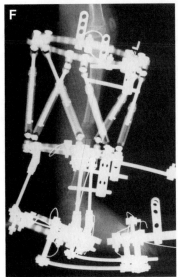

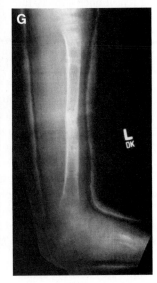

Fig. 3. Patient who has fibular hemimelia and a significant equinus and cavus foot deformity. (*A*) Preoperative clinical photograph. (*B*) Lateral view radiograph shows midtibial procurvatum deformity with severe equinus and cavus deformities. (*C*) Postoperative lateral view radiograph after the Taylor spatial frame was applied. (*D*) Postoperative lateral view clinical photograph of the Taylor spatial frame. Note that this fixator uses the virtual hinge (constrained) method. (*E*) After the equinus deformity is corrected, the foot ring is cut (medial and lateral) to allow for correction of the cavus deformity. The gradual distraction is accomplished by adding pusher and puller Ilizarov rods. (*F*) Lateral view radiograph of the cavus deformity correction. (*G*) Postoperative lateral view radiograph shows a plantigrade foot in a short-leg bivalved cast brace. The cast brace is worn for several months to maintain correction.

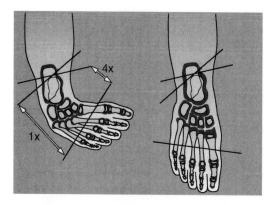

Fig. 4. Forefoot adduction correction with an Ilizarov apparatus (4:1 adjustment ratio medial to lateral, respectively) in a child allows for anatomic formation of cartilage and bone.

Ilizarov distraction is the preferred method to treat clubfoot with severe relapse after surgical treatment. These feet show extensive scar-tissue formation, and performing repeat open surgery through the scar is a daunting task. With Ilizarov techniques, the foot should be overcorrected by 5° to 10° in the plane of correction because of a tendency for the deformity to recur. It should be held in the overcorrected position for 4 to 6 weeks. After removal, a long leg cast is applied to maintain the overcorrected position. A custom-molded ankle-foot orthotic should be worn for the first 6 months. If dynamic recurrence is experienced, then the appropriate tendon transfer should be considered. Rigid recurrences might require appropriate corrective osteotomies with arthrodesis.

Toe flexion contractures commonly occur during correction and often are caused by tightening of the intrinsic and extrinsic toe flexors. To prevent toe flexion contractures, the toes should be stretched with toe slings made from leather and elastic bands or with a molded toe splint held to the fixator with Velcro straps. In addition, regular physical therapy is required to prevent toe stiffness and contractures. For preexisting toe contractures, consider percutaneous flexor tenotomy at the plantar digital crease. In older children, toe wires can be used to gradually pull the toes upward or maintain a corrected digital position (Fig. 5).

In the immature skeleton, spontaneous fracture through the distal tibial physis can occur during distraction. Physiolysis can be avoided by inserting a transverse wire into the distal tibial epiphysis connected to the tibial frame to stabilize the growth plate (Fig. 6).

The Ilizarov apparatus and Taylor spatial frame can also be used in conjunction with the principles described by Ponseti [19] for correction of recurrent clubfoot deformity. The forefoot position can be improved before surgery by a brief period of preoperative casting to allow for a less complicated frame construct. In the Ponseti sequence, the foot is first externally rotated through the subtalar joint. The initial correction with the Taylor spatial frame is programmed

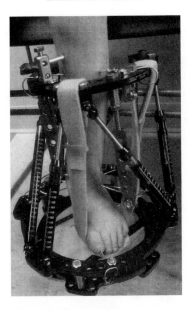

Fig. 5. Custom-molded forefoot plate with Velcro straps assists in the prevention of digital flexion contractures during deformity correction of the foot and ankle. Digital pinning can also be performed to correct or prevent toe flexion contractures.

for external rotation, valgus correction, and minimal dorsiflexion. A lateral olive wire through the talar neck mimics the thumb that Ponseti uses for counter-pressure. This wire is attached to the proximal tibial ring. After the foot is externally rotated approximately 40°, the talus neck olive wire is connected to the foot ring to allow for dorsiflexion of the ankle. Next, an additional program is created to allow for ankle dorsiflexion and the position is maintained to hold the correction (Fig. 7). This method is similar to the method used by Joshi [20], who developed an inexpensive, simple external fixator for clubfoot correction. This investigator emphasized correcting the varus deformity with distraction and then equinus correction. This unconstrained device permits the external rotation to occur. This rationale can be explained as follows: unconstrained external rotation of the calcaneal-pedal block allows for normal subtalar joint motion about its axis. Therefore, the calcaneal-pedal block's external rotation allows for talus-foot realignment. After the normal calcaneal talus relationship is restored, the ankle can be safely dorsiflexed. The combined subtalar and ankle joint motion is called *kinematic coupling* [19].

Arthrogryposis, teratologic clubfoot

Many congenital syndromes cause severe foot deformities. For example, arthrogryposis can cause patients to experience severe clubfoot contractures that

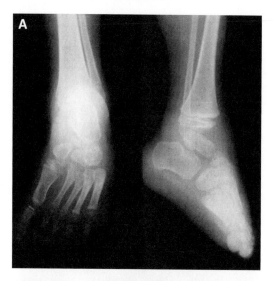

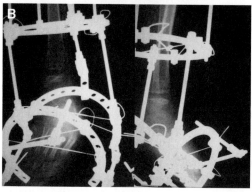

Fig. 6. Physiolysis or distraction of the growth plate can occur when deformity correction is being performed about the foot and ankle. (*A*) Preoperative anteroposterior view (*left*) and lateral view (*right*) radiographs of the left ankle. (*B*) Postoperative anteroposterior view (*left*) and lateral view (*right*) radiographs of the left ankle. Note the radiographic distraction of the distal tibial physis.

are associated with a high rate of recurrence after treatment. Treatment with external fixation using soft tissue and joint distraction in young children and distraction through osteotomies combined with joint arthrodesis in older children is a reasonable alternative for these severe, stiff, and often multiply operated feet [21,22].

Recurrences in children with arthrogryposis are common and might require subsequent correction in the form of arthrodesis or osteotomy (Fig. 8). In such cases, the authors generally perform extensive open surgery for acute correction of the hindfoot and ankle deformity. The external fixator is then applied for simultaneous tibial lengthening and static fixation of the foot correction.

Osteotomy

The primary indication for correction through bone is a fixed bony deformity. In patients younger than 8 years, some remodeling can still be expected and attempts at joint distraction are reasonable. When bony deformity is present in patients older than 8 years, soft tissue releases and distractions have a high rate

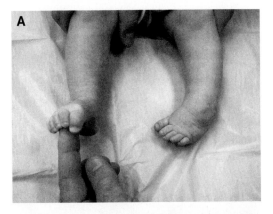

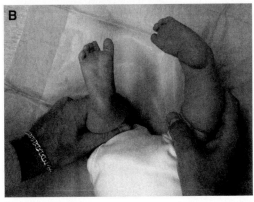

Fig. 7. Relapsed clubfoot. (*A*, *B*) Clinical photographs obtained when the infant initially presented. The photographs show the equinus and varus deformity of the left hindfoot and the adduction and supination deformity of the left forefoot. (*C*) Lateral view radiograph shows the residual clubfoot in the 8-year-old child. (*D*) Anteroposterior view radiograph shows the residual clubfoot in the 8-year-old child. (*E*) Intraoperative fluoroscopy shows an olive wire inserted from lateral to medial through the talar neck. Note the distal tibial epiphysial stirrup wire, which prevents physiolysis. The left panel shows a lateral view of the ankle and the right panel shows an anteroposterior view of the ankle. (*F*) Postoperative photograph shows the talar neck wire attached to the tibial ring by way of plates. (*G*) Clinical photograph shows the completion of the first stage of treatment (foot external rotation). When the foot is externally rotated 40°, the dorsiflexion of the ankle can begin. (*H*) Clinical photograph of the anteroposterior view of the foot. Note that the talar wire was detached from the tibial ring (plates removed) and reattached to the foot ring. (*I*) Lateral view radiograph of the foot. The ankle can now be safely dorsiflexed. (*J*) Lateral view clinical photograph of the foot. (*K*) Final postoperative lateral view radiograph shows a plantigrade foot position.

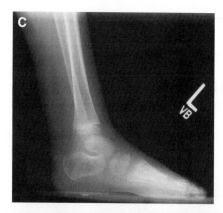

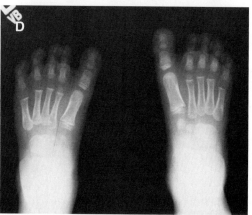

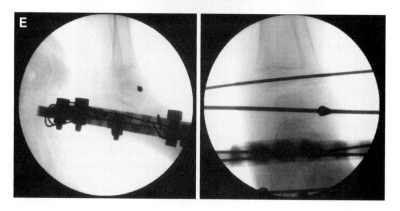

Fig. 7 (*continued*).

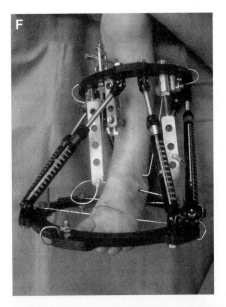

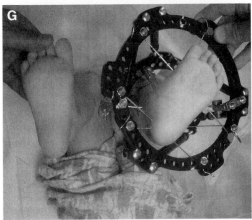

Fig. 7 (*continued*).

of recurrence. Other indications for an osteotomy include neuromuscular imbalance. Occasionally, it is not possible to maintain correction obtained by distraction. In such cases, arthrodesis can be considered with osteotomy. Nonunion,
the presence of previous fusions, and severe stiffness of deformities are also
indications for osseous correction [17,23]. Osteotomy provides osseous realignment with acute or gradual correction by way of external fixation or acute correction with internal fixation.

Supramalleolar osteotomies are indicated for deformities of the metaphysial
or juxta-articular region. Other indications include deformity at the level of a

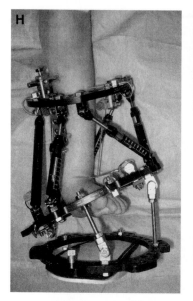
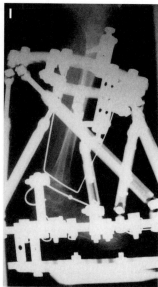

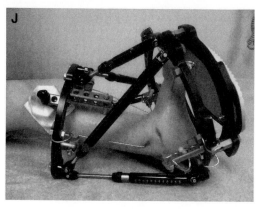

Fig. 7 (*continued*).

previous arthrodesis and deformities at the level of the talus or subtalar joint in the presence of ankle ankylosis. Equinus, calcaneus, varus, and valgus deformities and tibial torsion and limb-length discrepancies can be corrected through the metaphysial or juxta-articular region. The level of the osteotomy (within 2.5 cm of the ankle joint) is critical for providing reliable bone consolidation. In addition, the method with which the osteotomy is performed is important for bone formation; the authors prefer the percutaneous Gigli saw technique through the tibia and fibula [7]. Supramalleolar osteotomy with external fixation allows for gradual correction of length, angulation, translation, and rotation. Although the procedure avoids performing surgery on a foot that has undergone multiple

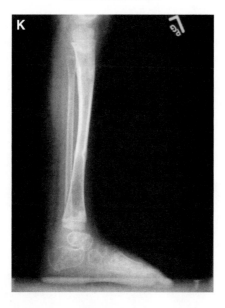

Fig. 7 (*continued*).

operations, it does not allow correction of deformities between the hindfoot and forefoot. When the level of deformity is at a level different from that of the osteotomy, translation is required to prevent the creation of a secondary deformity (see Fig. 8).

The U osteotomy passes under the subtalar joint through the superior part of the calcaneus posteriorly and across the sinus tarsi and neck of the talus anteriorly. It is indicated when the deformity occurs in the talus, such as in a case of flattop talus. The foot can be repositioned into a plantigrade position while leaving the ankle mortise undisturbed. Although this osteotomy can be performed acutely, most deformities require gradual realignment with the external fixator. The U osteotomy crosses the sinus tarsi and physically blocks the subtalar joint; therefore, it should not be performed in a patient who has normal subtalar motion. The U osteotomy can correct foot height and equinus, calcaneus, varus, and valgus deformities. It is unable to correct deformities between the hindfoot and forefoot (Fig. 9) [7].

The V osteotomy is a double osteotomy. One osteotomy crosses the body of the calcaneus posterior to the subtalar joint, and the other crosses the midfoot at the neck of the talus and calcaneus through the sinus tarsi, the cuboid-navicular row, or the cuboid-cuneiform row. When the midfoot osteotomy is made across the neck of the talus and calcaneus, it converges with the posterior calcaneal osteotomy on the plantar aspect of the calcaneus. The procedure leaves a triangular wedge of calcaneus and subtalar joint connected by the posterior facet to the body of the talus. The triangular wedge must be fixed in place during distraction. This type of V osteotomy is indicated when deformities are present between the forefoot and hindfoot with an associated stiff subtalar joint. When preservation of the subtalar joint motion is important, the anterior segment of the V should be made through the cuboid-navicular or cuboid-cuneiform rows. Hindfoot and forefoot osteotomies can correct all types of foot deformities, including hindfoot and forefoot equinus or calcaneus deformities, rockerbottom deformities, cavus deformities, abductus or adductus deformities, supination

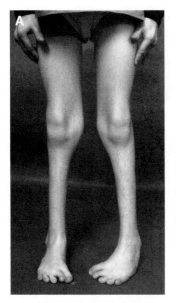
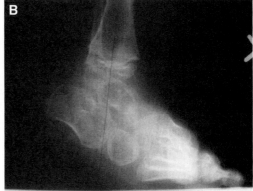

Fig. 8. Arthrogryposis. (*A*) Clinical photograph shows a case of severe clubfoot. The right limb presents with significant internal tibial torsion and forefoot varus deformity. The left limb presents with ankle equinus and ankle varus deformities. (*B*) Lateral view radiograph shows the residual forefoot varus deformity, supination deformity of the hindfoot, and equinus deformity in the right limb. (*C*) Lateral view radiograph of the left limb is similar to that of the right limb, but the left limb presents with a more severe equinus deformity. (*D*) Anteroposterior view radiographs of bilateral feet show forefoot abduction and supination. (*E*) Intraoperative fluoroscopy shows a midfoot osteotomy performed on the right foot (*left*) and a supramalleolar osteotomy performed on the left tibia using the percutaneous Gigli saw technique (*right*). (*F*) Postoperative clinical photograph shows the patient after the application of bilateral external fixators. (*G*) Lateral view radiograph shows that the right forefoot is first distracted on a fixed hindfoot. (*H*) After gradually distracting the forefoot (1.5 cm), the patient returns to the operating room for the second stage of the procedure. The forefoot threaded rods are removed. (*I*) During the second stage of the procedure, the forefoot is also pronated acutely to a neutral position and held in the new position by replacing the threaded rods. (*J*) Supramalleolar osteotomy performed on the left limb corrects the foot as a unit from a varus deformity to a neutral hindfoot to tibial relationship. (*K*) Lateral view radiograph shows a plantigrade foot position after correction with the supramalleolar osteotomy. (*L*) Final postoperative lateral view radiograph of the right limb shows a plantigrade foot position. (*M*) Final postoperative lateral view radiograph of the left limb shows a plantigrade foot position.

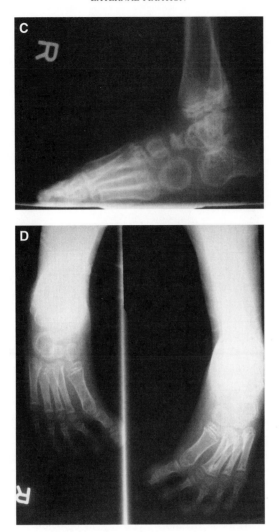

Fig. 8 (*continued*).

deformities, pronation deformities, and even bony deficiency of the hindfoot or forefoot. Again, this procedure is performed as a gradual correction with the use of external fixation [7]. As an alternative, the same approach can be performed with closing wedge correction of one or both osteotomies using internal or external fixation.

The posterior calcaneal osteotomy is essentially the posterior segment of the V osteotomy. It is used in cases of isolated deformities of the hindfoot and can be combined with soft tissue correction of the forefoot. Posterior calcaneal osteotomies are performed acutely with pin or screw fixation and include the

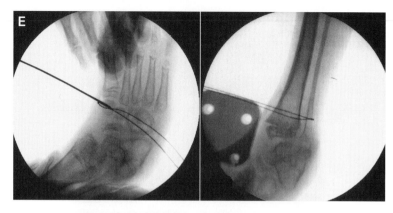

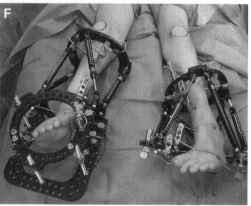

Fig. 8 (*continued*).

Dwyer (closing lateral wedge), medial, lateral, dorsal, and plantar displacement osteotomies. The dorsal opening wedge osteotomy, however, is typically performed through gradual distraction, especially in complex realignment cases. Calcaneal bone deficiency due to congenital or posttraumatic causes can be treated by lengthening of the calcaneus through this osteotomy. Smooth wires or half-pins can be inserted through the posterior calcaneal segment for fixation. Smooth wires and half-pins can cut through or pull out of the calcaneus as the calcaneus becomes osteoporotic during the treatment period; therefore, careful postoperative monitoring is important. Ilizarov hinges should be placed at the apex of the angular correction and, with the Taylor spatial frame, appropriate planning of a dorsally opening wedge osteotomy should be performed. In a short or stubby calcaneus, distraction of the calcaneal tuber in a posterior direction provides a greater lever arm for the Achilles tendon and prevents the heel from slipping up out of the shoe.

The talocalcaneal neck osteotomy is essentially the anterior segment of the V osteotomy. It is used for correction of forefoot deformities in the presence of a

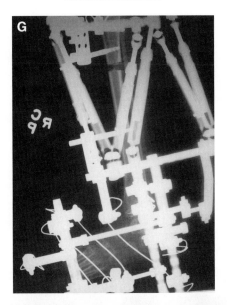

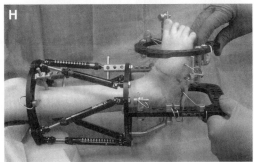

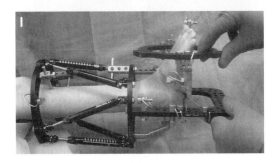

Fig. 8 (*continued*).

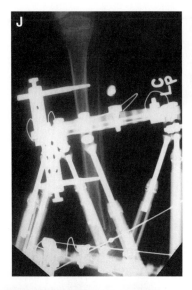
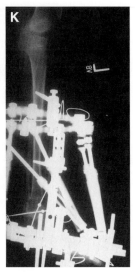
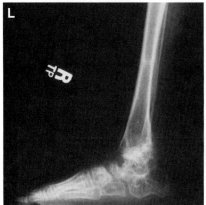
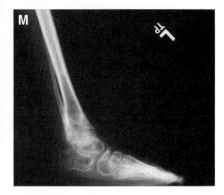

Fig. 8 (*continued*).

stiff or ankylosed subtalar joint. When a mobile subtalar joint is present, a midfoot osteotomy across the cuboid and navicular bones or across the cuboid bone and cuneiforms should be used.

The authors prefer to perform all three midfoot-type osteotomies using the percutaneous Gigli saw technique [7]. The Gigli saw should never be used to perform osteotomies across multiple metatarsals because of risk of neurovascular injury. A midfoot osteotomy can also be used to lengthen the midfoot. For a foot with normal mobile joints, a midfoot osteotomy is associated with a high risk of creating a stiff foot. In cases in which the foot is already stiff, the authors advise against lengthening the midfoot.

Metatarsal lengthening

Lengthening for short metatarsals is best delayed until skeletal maturity; however, metatarsal lengthening can be performed in children who have severe deformities and length discrepancies and deficiencies, as long as the growth centers are preserved. Gradual lengthening with external fixation is preferred for metatarsal lengthening greater than 1 cm [24]. With gradual lengthening, the rate of postoperative lengthening can be adjusted and the patient can bear weight during treatment. Unlike acute lengthening, which can cause severe soft tissue stretch, gradual lengthening reduces the risk of neurovascular compromise [24,25]. Lengthening of short metatarsals has been performed with an acute

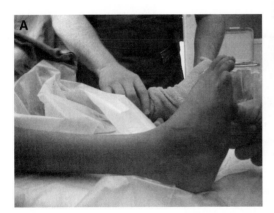
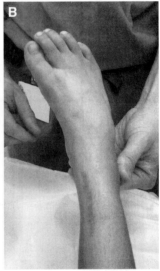

Fig. 9. Residual clubfoot. (*A*) Clinical photograph shows a clubfoot that has undergone previous operations and is stiff. Note the equinus deformity. (*B*) Clinical photograph shows the forefoot abduction. (*C*) Clinical photograph shows the combined forefoot and hindfoot varus deformity. (*D*) Anteroposterior view radiograph shows normal ankle alignment. (*E*) Long standing, lateral view radiograph of the foot and ankle shows cavovarus deformity. (*F*) Long standing, calcaneal axial radiograph shows significant hindfoot varus. (*G*) A foot board is used intraoperatively to confirm the diagnosis of a combined forefoot and hindfoot varus deformity. (*H*) Fluoroscopy shows the multiple osteotome technique used to perform the U osteotomy, which is made beneath the sustentaculum tali and through the neck of the talus. (*I*) Under fluoroscopy, the osteotomy is visualized to ensure completion. (*J*, *K*) Postoperative clinical photographs show the limb after application of a Taylor spatial frame. (*L*) Postoperative anteroposterior view radiograph. (*M*) Postoperative lateral view radiograph. (*N*) Clinical photograph obtained after correction shows how the U osteotomy corrects the foot as a unit. Note the neutral heel position. (*O*) Clinical photograph shows the external rotation of the foot. (*P*) Clinical photograph shows a plantigrade position of the foot. (*Q*) Lateral view radiograph shows that the foot is in a plantigrade position after removal of the external fixator.

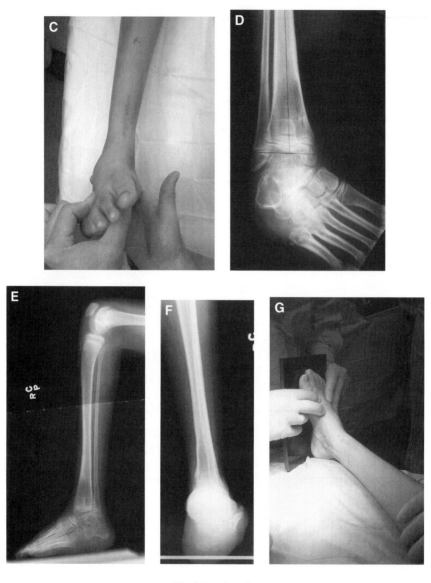

Fig. 9 (*continued*).

interpositional bone graft or by distraction osteogenesis [26]. The authors prefer a monolateral, mini external fixator for metatarsal lengthening even when multiple metatarsals are lengthened simultaneously. Distraction is performed at a rate of 0.5 mm per day divided into 0.25-mm increments. It is important that the plane and vector of metatarsal lengthening be such that the final position of the

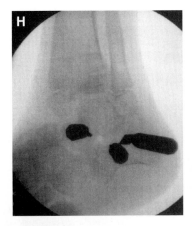

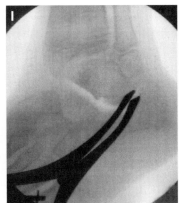

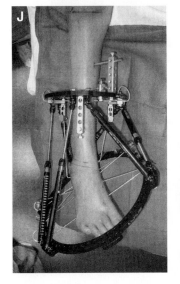

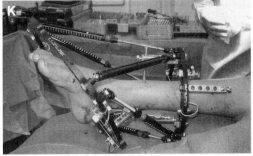

Fig. 9 (*continued*).

metatarsal head is located at the appropriate level in the sagittal and transverse planes, respectively. Pinning of the metatarsal phalangeal joint is recommended to prevent subluxation or contracture of the toe (Fig. 10).

Tibial lengthening

Patients who have foot and ankle deformities often present with concurrent limb-length discrepancies. Limb-length discrepancy can be congential, traumatic,

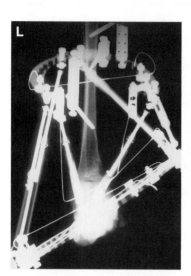

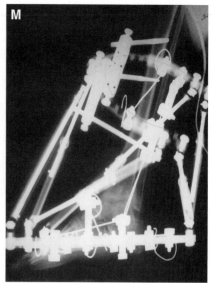

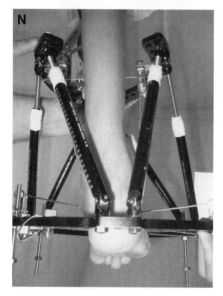

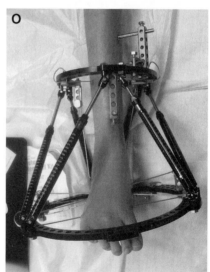

Fig. 9 (*continued*).

or secondary to previous surgery, arthrodesis, or malalignment. Limb lengthening is a challenging procedure that demands an experienced surgeon. Most tibial lengthenings are performed proximally through a proximal metaphysial corticotomy or Gigli saw osteotomy. Fixation of the tibia and the fibula is important to avoid descent of the fibula or proximal migration of the distal fibula. When

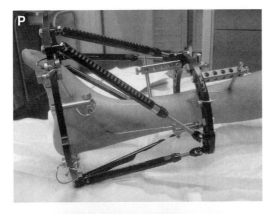

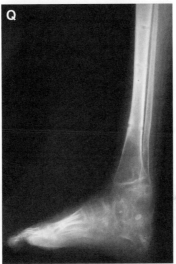

Fig. 9 (*continued*).

applying a fixator to the proximal tibia, care should be taken to avoid injury to the common peroneal nerve. Distal tibial lengthening is performed when a deformity is present at or proximal to the ankle joint. To prevent equinus deformity, the external fixator should be extended to the foot for distal tibial, double-level, and longer lengthenings.

Ankle equinus and knee contractures are common problems that can arise with lengthening. A 5-day-per-week combined land and aquatic physical therapy regimen is critical to avoid these joint contractures. In addition, dynamic knee and ankle extension splints can be used. A prophylactic gastrocnemius-soleus recession can be performed in the case of a high-risk patient or a preoperative equinus contracture. Axial deviation, such as an osseous deformity, can occur during lengthening. This deviation occurs secondary to the surrounding posterior and lateral muscle mass about the tibia. When the amount of tension is high enough, the bone deviates in the direction of the larger muscle mass. In the proximal tibia, procurvatum and valgus deformities together with lateral and

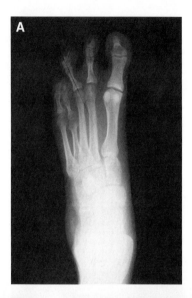

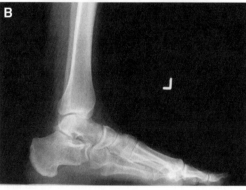

Fig. 10. Congenital short fourth metatarsal lengthening. (*A*) Anteroposterior view radiograph shows a slight medial bowing of the fourth metatarsal. (*B*) Preoperative lateral view radiograph shows an increased fourth metatarsal declination and an extension contracture of the toe. The increased declination is observed at the level of the distal metaphysial-diaphysial junction (the region of the growth plate). Note that the dorsal cortex of the short metatarsal is parallel to the adjacent metatarsals. (*C*) Anteroposterior view radiograph shows that pinning the digit across the metatarsophalangeal joint prevents digital dislocation and that mounting the pin to the fixator prevents pin dislodgement during lengthening. (*D*) Oblique radiographic view of the foot shows normotrophic formation of regenerated bone in the fourth metatarsal. (*E*) Postoperative anteroposterior view radiograph. (*F*) Postoperative lateral view radiograph.

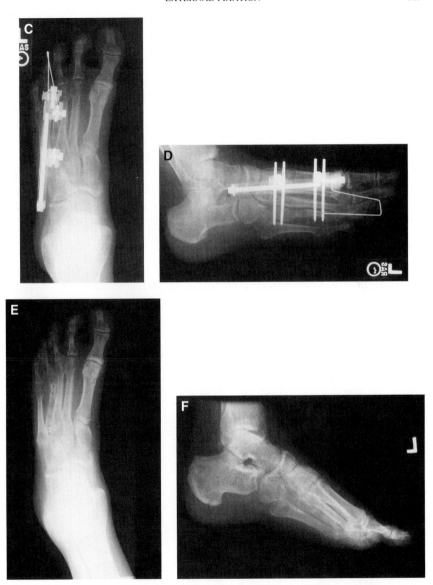

Fig. 10 (*continued*).

posterior translation, respectively, can occur and increase in severity with increased amounts of tibial lengthening. Alignment should be assessed by using the appropriate long standing radiographs during treatment. In the case of an unstable ankle joint or a ball-and-socket ankle joint, it is important to fix the foot with lateral opposing olive wires [27].

Acute trauma

External fixation is an important tool for surgeons treating distal tibial, foot, and ankle trauma. These injuries are often associated with soft tissue compromise, especially in cases of open fracture and crush injury. External fixation can be used as a temporary splint to allow for reduction of soft tissue swelling before definitive internal fixation or as a neutralization device combined with internal fixation to maintain axial alignment and hold a correction [28,29]. High-energy injuries and injuries with compromised skin lend themselves well to correction by external fixation because the method causes limited soft tissue disruption. External fixation provides stability to multiple bone segments, allowing access and healing of soft tissue wounds without compromising the bone healing. Modern external fixation devices allow for acute or gradual reduction of the fracture. Another advantage of external fixation includes the prevention of soft tissue contractures [30].

In most pediatric cases, fractures are typically treated with casts; however, in cases that involve complex distal tibial fractures, external fixation is an excellent tool to treat children and adolescents. The Taylor spatial frame or Ilizarov apparatus allows for gradual or acute reduction in fractures that cannot be controlled with casting techniques (Fig. 11). External fixation can also be used in

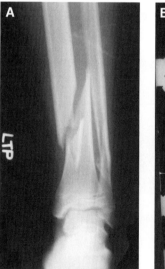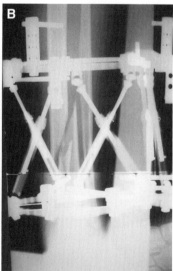

Fig. 11. Distal tibiofibular fracture. (*A*) Preoperative anteroposterior view radiograph shows a comminuted distal tibiofibular fracture. (*B*) Postoperative anteroposterior view radiograph shows the Taylor spatial frame and the distal tibial malalignment. (*C*) Anteroposterior view radiograph shows the anatomic alignment after gradual correction with the external fixator. (*D*) Anteroposterior view radiograph shows a healed, aligned distal tibia and fibula after removal of the external fixator.

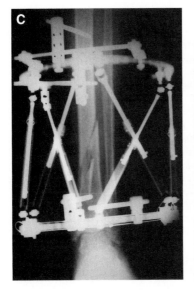
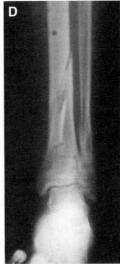

Fig. 11 (*continued*).

the treatment of complex midfoot, tarsal, and metatarsal injury fractures, particularly in association with severe soft tissue injuries.

Summary

External fixation has many applications to the pediatric foot and ankle. Additional applications of external fixation continue to be developed as technology and experience improve. External fixation should not be performed by a surgeon inexperienced in the technique. It is vital to gain knowledge from courses, lectures, seminars, and books about the topic. Surgeons who wish to use external fixation should visit and observe at centers where external fixation is frequently performed and obtain personal instruction from surgeons experienced in the Ilizarov method.

References

[1] Paley D, Herzenberg JE. Applications of external fixation to foot and ankle reconstruction. In: Myerson MS, editor. Foot and ankle disorders, vol. 2. Philadelphia: WB Saunders; 2000. p. 1135–88.

[2] Herzenberg JE, Paley D. Ilizarov applications in foot and ankle surgery. Adv Orthop Surg 1992;16(3):162–74.

[3] Codivilla A. On the means of lengthening in the lower limbs, the muscles and tissues which are shortened through deformity. Am J Orthop Surg 1905;2:353–63.

[4] Paley D. Current techniques of limb lengthening. J Pediatr Orthop 1988;8(1):73–92.

[5] [No authors listed]. Kurgan revolution in orthopedics. J Am Podiatry Assoc 1973;63(12):687–8.

[6] LaBianco GJ, Vito GR, Kalish SR. Use of the Ilizarov external fixator in the treatment of lower extremity deformities. J Am Podiatr Med Assoc 1996;86(11):523–31.

[7] Paley D. Principles of deformity correction. Berlin: Springer-Verlag; 2002.

[8] Calhoun JH, Burke-Evans E, Herndon DN. Techniques for the management of burn contractures with the Ilizarov fixator. Clin Orthop 1992;280:117–24.

[9] Erdoğan B, Gorgu M, Girgin O, et al. Application of external fixators in major foot contractures. J Foot Ankle Surg 1996;35(3):218–21.

[10] Lamm BM, Paley D, Herzenberg JE. Gastrocnemius soleus recession: a simpler, more limited approach. J Am Podiatr Med Assoc 2005;95(1):18–25.

[11] Bassett GS, Mazur KU, Sloan GM. Soft tissue expander failure in severe equinovarus foot deformity. J Pediatr Orthop 1993;13(6):744–8.

[12] Ohmori S. Correction of burn deformities using free flap transfer. J Trauma 1982;22(2):104–11.

[13] Paley D. The correction of complex foot deformities using Ilizarov's distraction osteotomies. Clin Orthop 1993;293:97–111.

[14] Paley D. Principles of foot deformity correction: Ilizarov technique. In: Gould JS, editor. Operative foot surgery. Philadelphia: WB Saunders; 1994. p. 476–514.

[15] Franke J, Grill F, Hein G, et al. Correction of clubfoot relapse using Ilizarov's apparatus in children 8–15 years old. Arch Orthop Trauma Surg 1990;110(1):33–7.

[16] Grill F, Franke J. The Ilizarov distractor for the correction of relapsed or neglected clubfoot. J Bone Joint Surg Br 1987;69(4):593–7.

[17] Reinker KA, Carpenter CT. Ilizarov applications in the pediatric foot. J Pediatr Orthop 1997; 17(6):796–802.

[18] Wallander H, Hansson G, Tjernström B. Correction of persistent clubfoot deformities with the Ilizarov external fixator. Acta Orthop Scand 1996;67(3):283–7.

[19] Ponseti IV. Congenital clubfoot: fundamentals of treatment. New York: Oxford University Press; 1996.

[20] Joshi BB. Correction of congenital talipes equino varus (CTEV) by controlled differential fractional distraction using Joshi's external stabilization system (JESS). 1st edition. Mumbai, India: JESS Research and Development Centre; 2001.

[21] Huang SC. Soft tissue contractures of the knee or ankle treated by the Ilizarov technique. Acta Orthop Scand 1996;67(5):443–9.

[22] Brunner R, Hefti F, Tgetgel JD. Arthrogrypotic joint contracture at the knee and foot: correction with a circular frame. J Pediatr Orthop B 1997;6(3):192–7.

[23] Grant AD, Atar D, Lehman WB. Ilizarov technique in correction of foot deformities: a preliminary report. Foot Ankle 1990;11(1):1–5.

[24] Davidson RS. Metatarsal lengthening. Foot Ankle Clin 2001;6(3):499–518.

[25] Levine SE, Davidson RS, Dormans JP, et al. Distraction osteogenesis for congenitally short lesser metatarsals. Foot Ankle Int 1995;16(4):196–200.

[26] Choudhury SN, Kitaoka HB, Peterson HA. Metatarsal lengthening: case report and review of literature. Foot Ankle Int 1997;18(11):739–45.

[27] Paley D, Kovelman HF, Herzenberg JE. Ilizarov technology. In: Stauffer RN, editor. Advances in operative orthopaedics, vol. 1. St. Louis (MO): Mosby-Year Book; 1993. p. 243–87.

[28] Seibert FJ, Fankhauser F, Elliott B, et al. External fixation in trauma of the foot and ankle. Clin Podiatr Med Surg 2003;20(1):159–80.

[29] Aktuglu K, Ozsoy MH, Yensel U. Treatment of displaced pylon fractures with circular external fixators of Ilizarov. Foot Ankle Int 1998;19(4):208–16.

[30] Kenzora JE, Edwards CC, Browner BD, et al. Acute management of major trauma involving the foot and ankle with Hoffman external fixation. Foot Ankle 1981;1(6):348–61.

ELSEVIER
SAUNDERS

Clin Podiatr Med Surg
23 (2006) 167–189

CLINICS IN
PODIATRIC
MEDICINE AND
SURGERY

Fractures and Dislocations of the Foot in Children

Johannes Mayr, MD[a],*, Gerolf Peicha, MD[b],
Wolfgang Grechenig, MD[b], Randolf Hammerl, MD[c],
Andreas Weiglein, MD[d], Erich Sorantin, MD[e]

[a]*Department of Pediatric Surgery, University Children's Hospital Basle (UKBB), Postbox,
4005 Basle, Switzerland*
[b]*Department of Trauma, Medical University Graz, Auenbruggerplatz 39, A–8036 Graz, Austria*
[c]*Department of Internal Medicine, Federal Hospital Fuerstenfeld, Styria, Austria*
[d]*Institute of Anatomy, Medical University Graz, Harrachgasse 21, A–8010 Graz, Austria*
[e]*Division of Paediatric Radiology, Department of Radiology, Medical University Graz,
Auenbruggerplatz 34, A–8036 Graz, Austria*

Foot fractures account for 12% of all pediatric fractures. Toe fractures are more frequently observed in children aged 11 to 15 years, whereas other foot fractures are more frequently seen in children aged 0 to 6 years. Dislocations of foot joints are extremely rare in children. Foot and ankle sprains account for 4.8% of all pediatric injuries, and foot and ankle contusions account for 3.9% of pediatric injuries. The distribution of foot and ankle injuries is shown in Table 1.

The challenge of managing pediatric foot injuries is the identification of the rare injuries that require operative treatment and the management of complications such as compartment syndrome, post-traumatic foot deformities, and avascular necrosis.

Fractures of the talus

Approximately two thirds of the surface of the talus is covered by articular cartilage [1]. Most fractures of the talus in children involve the talar neck. Forced

---

* Corresponding author.
E-mail address: mayrjm@gmx.at (J. Mayr).

0891-8422/06/$ – see front matter © 2006 Elsevier Inc. All rights reserved.
doi:10.1016/j.cpm.2005.10.011   *podiatric.theclinics.com*

Table 1
Distribution of foot and ankle injuries in children younger than age 16 years treated at the Department
of Pediatric Surgery during a 4-year interval

Type and location of injury	No. of children injured (%)
Injuries of all body regions	42,704 (100.0)
Fractures of all body regions	9481 (22.2)
Ankle fracture	350 (0.8)
Calcanal, talus, tarsal, metatarsal fracture	369 (0.9)
Toe fracture	774 (1.8)
Foot and ankle dislocation	19 (0.04)
Foot and ankle sprain	2031 (4.8)
Foot and ankle contusion	1680 (3.9)
Foot and ankle crushing injury	88 (0.2)

dorsiflexion of the foot in the ankle joint creates a concentration of deforming
force at the dorsal aspect of the talar neck, resulting in a fracture of the neck
(Fig. 1A). Talar neck fractures do not usually involve the articular surface of the
talus (see Fig. 1B); however, a crushing injury to the articular cartilage at the
anterior rim of the distal tibia may occur. Most talar neck fractures in children run
across the dorsal neck circumference to the region of the interosseous ligament.

Blood supply of the talus and risk of avascular necrosis

The head of the talus receives its blood supply from branches of the
perforating peroneal artery by way of the artery of the tarsal sinus, from branches
of the dorsalis pedis artery (Fig. 2), and from small arteries from the deltoid

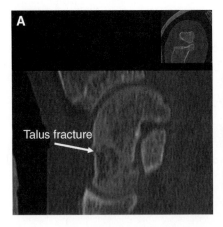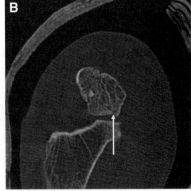

Fig. 1. (A) CT scan of an undisplaced, impacted, stable fracture of the talar neck sustained in a traffic
accident by a 14-year-old boy. (B) Minimal impression of the articular surface of the talus by the
sustentaculum tali of the calcaneus.

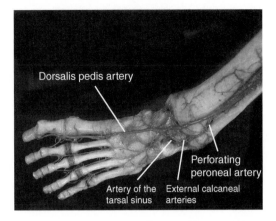

Fig. 2. Dorsal view of the arterial blood supply of the talus and forefoot. The artery of the tarsal sinus receives the blood supply for the head of the talus from branches of the perforating peroneal artery and dorsalis pedis artery.

branch of the posterior tibial artery (Fig. 3). The neck of the talus is the major entry point for the vascular supply to the head and body of the talus. The neck and corpus of the talus receive their blood supply from tarsal sinus branches of the perforating peroneal artery and branches of the dorsalis pedis artery; most of the blood supply comes from the artery of the tarsal canal, both branches of the posterior tibial artery, and the deltoid branch [2]. Basic knowledge of the vascular supply is mandatory to understand the risk of avascular necrosis caused by talar fractures [3,4].

A typical clinical sign of talar fractures is a circumscribed tenderness and swelling just above the talar neck in the anterior aspect of the ankle joint (Fig. 4). Displaced fractures caused by forced dorsiflexion in the ankle joint can be

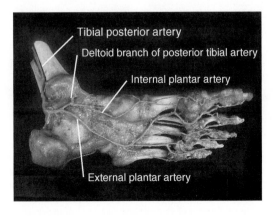

Fig. 3. Arteries from the deltoid branch of the posterior tibial artery supply the medial part of the talus.

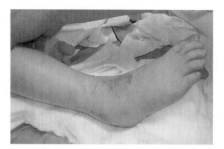

Fig. 4. Swelling and hematoma at the region above the talar neck in a 14-year-old boy who sustained an undisplaced talar neck fracture and a displaced calcaneal fracture in a rollover injury from a heavy machine.

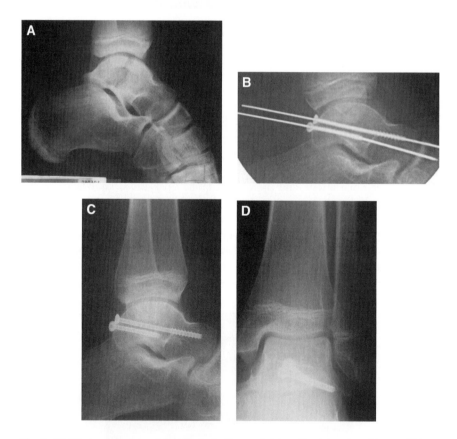

Fig. 5. (*A*) Displaced fracture of the talar body from a skateboarding injury in a 14-year-old boy. (*B*) Closed reduction and percutaneous fixation using two canulated screws (diameter 4.0 mm). (*C*) At 3 months postoperatively, the fracture has healed; however, there is 10° of plantarflexion restriction. (*D*) Anteroposterior view shows a subchondral lucency at the peroneal aspect of the corpus tali (positive Hawkins sign). (*E*) At the time of implant removal 6 months postoperatively, only one screw could be removed due to overgrowth of cartilage over the head of the second screw and problems turning the titanium screw backward.

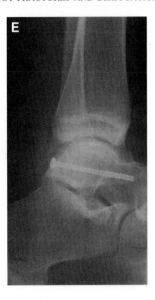

Fig. 5 (*continued*).

reduced by plantarflexion of the foot. Nowadays, only anterior and lateral radiographs are performed, with the beam centered on the hind foot. If possible, MRI or CT scans should be obtained (see Fig. 1A). The treatment of talar fractures in children is similar to that in adults. In older children, who are able to walk on crutches, a below-knee plaster cast is applied for 6 to 8 weeks, and non–weight bearing is recommended during this period. In younger children, who are unable to use crutches for non–weight bearing, a below-knee cast or a long leg cast with the knee flexed is applied for 4 to 6 weeks, depending on the stability and type of fracture and the age of the child. After consolidation of the fracture, a short leg, weight-bearing cast is applied for another 2 weeks. The authors recommend closed reduction and fixation by two small cannulated screws (diameter 3–4 mm) in displaced fractures of the talus. Reduction is necessary when the gap at the joint surface is 2 mm or more with an angulation greater than 15° (Fig. 5). In rare cases, a stable position of the talar neck fracture is obtained after closed reduction by plantarflexion of the foot. These fractures can be treated by applying a plaster cast in plantarflexed position, especially in the younger children. Follow-up radiographs are mandatory to check the correct reduction of the fracture.

For open reduction of talar neck fractures, a posterior or dorsomedial approach is used. Using the posterior approach, the insertion of screws lateral to the Achilles tendon is simple; however, fixation removal can be very demanding and should not be done unless there is some striking indication (see Fig. 5E). When using the dorsomedial approach, care must be taken to enter the soft tissues medial to the extensor hallucis longus tendon to prevent injury to the dorsalis pedis artery and deep peroneal nerve. Follow-up of talus fractures in children should continue for at least 3 years. Avascular necrosis is the most serious complication of talar fractures in children; the occurrence of this complication mainly depends on the type of fracture and the initial displacement (Figs. 6 and 7). It should be noted that avascular necrosis of the talus can occur even in undisplaced fractures of the talus. Development of avascular necrosis of the talus does not depend on the time elapsed from injury to reduction or on the age of the child [5].

Classification of fractures according to Marti [6] (Table 2) does not influence the initial treatment; however, a prolonged period of partial weight bearing up to 6 months after the injury in cases carrying a high risk of avascular necrosis is advisable. The authors recommend physical therapy to prevent restriction of ankle joint range of motion until a normal gait pattern is evident. The classification according to Marti [6] assesses the risk of avascular necrosis in any particular fracture of the talus in children. Undisplaced fractures of the talus carry a low risk of avascular necrosis compared with displaced fractures. The Hawkins sign (an area of subchondral lucency in the dome of the talus) is a sign of viability of the talar body after fracture (see Fig. 5D). It was found that this line could be absent in children who sustained nondisplaced talar fractures and had short periods of non–weight bearing or immobilization [7]. Nowadays, fractures of the talus should undergo MRI for the diagnosis of avascular necrosis in the first weeks after trauma; the findings influence the period of immobilization. Avascular necrosis of the talus in children can run a prolonged course but is usually well tolerated by children and their families. In children suffering post-

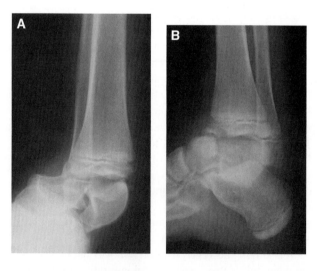

Fig. 6. (*A, B*) Displaced fracture of the neck of the talus, ankle joint dislocation, subtalar joint dislocation, and displaced Salter-Harris type III fracture of the medial malleolus in a 13-year-old boy who was tackled during American football training.

traumatic avascular necrosis of the talus, the authors allow full weight bearing 4 months after union of the fracture but recommend that the child refrains from jumping and participating in contact sports. The authors regularly repeat MRI studies (usually twice a year) to screen for loose bodies in the ankle joint within the first years after the injury. In the authors' opinion, surgical interventions in

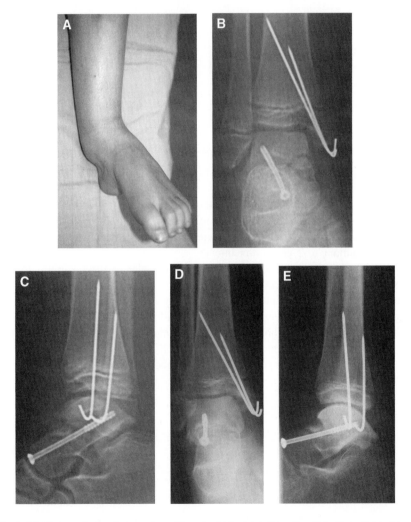

Fig. 7. (*A*) Photograph showing massive ankle and subtalar joint dislocation indicative of high risk of avascular necrosis of the talar body. (*B, C*) Intraoperative images taken during open reduction after fixation of talus fractures using 4.0-mm canulated screws and K-wire stabilization of the medial malleolus. (*D, E*) Two months after injury, there is a significant sclerosation of the talar body, indicative of subtotal avascular necrosis of the talar body (this finding was confirmed by MRI after removal of K-wires). (*F, G*) At 4 years postoperatively, flattening of the trochlea tali and arthrosis of the tibio talar joint are evident. Stiffness of the subtalar joint was also noted.

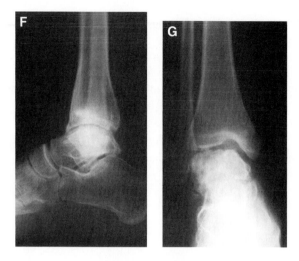

Fig. 7 (*continued*).

cases of avascular necrosis of the talus should be limited during the growth age to the extraction of loose intra-articular bodies residing within the ankle joint. The radiologic alterations of the ankle joint, however, can show prearthrosis or arthrosis within 1 to 2 years after injury.

Avulsion injuries of the lateral or posterior talar process can be treated conservatively in most cases, provided there is no gross displacement or interference with ankle joint movements. Only in rare cases, when there is a fragment of adequate size, is fixation by a small cannulated screw indicated.

The treatment of osteochondral ("flake") fractures of the trochlea tali depends on the initial displacement of the fragment (Fig. 8) [8–10]; however, it is necessary to discern these lesions from osteochondritis dissecans. Usually, the

Table 2
Classification of fractures of the talus according to Marti

Type	Fracture	Prognosis/blood supply	Risk of avascular necrosis
I	Distal neck	Talar blood supply intact	None
II	Undisplaced proximal neck or body fracture	Talar blood supply usually intact	Small
III	Displaced proximal neck or body fracture	Intraosseal blood circulation blocked, auxiliary blood supply intact	Significant
IV	Proximal neck with dislocation of the talus body outside the ankle joint	All blood supply to the talus blocked	100%

Data from Marti R. Fractures of the talus and calcaneus. In: Weber BG, Brunner C, Freuler F, editors. Treatment of fractures in children and adolescents. New York: Springer; 1980. p. 378.

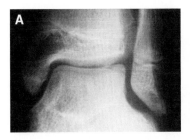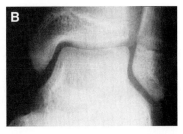

Fig. 8. (*A*) Undisplaced osteochondral "flake" fracture at the lateral circumference of the trochlea tali from a trampoline injury in a 12-year-old girl. Treatment included plaster cast immobilization for 6 weeks and limited weight bearing for another 6 weeks. (*B*) After 3 months, the osteochondral fracture has healed.

appearance of an osteochondritis dissecans lesion resembles an older lesion with rounded edges of the fragment, fragmentation of the fragment, and distinct sclerosis of the bed of the lesion. If possible, osteochondral fractures and osteochondritis dissecans should undergo MRI studies before treatment. Undisplaced osteochondral fractures can be treated by initial immobilization and non–weight bearing for at least 6 weeks and limited weight bearing for another 6 weeks. Before weight bearing is allowed, consolidation of the fracture should be confirmed by radiography or MRI. Displaced osteochondral fractures should preferably be treated arthroscopically. This approach can eliminate the need to do a medial malleolar osteotomy [11,12].

Subtalar dislocations are extremely rare in young children [13]. The largest series of five subtalar dislocations was described by Dimentberg and Rosman [14]. These injuries are sometimes difficult to diagnose by radiographs due to the presence of other injuries [14]. The authors observed one osseous ankylosis of the anterior subtalar joint in a boy who sustained a combined talus neck and central calcaneal fracture (Fig. 9). The boy suffered recurrent posterior subtalar joint effusions and recurrent pain in the posterior subtalar joint together with a blockage of subtalar joint movements [15].

Fractures of the calcaneus

Fractures of the calcaneus in children are rare but observed more frequently compared with fractures of the talus [16,17]. Most of these fractures are caused by falls from a height, from running, or from injuries caused by motor vehicles or heavy machines. Calcaneal fractures caused by a fall from a height are often accompanied by injuries of the spine. The secondary ossification center of the calcaneus in young children is oval shaped and surrounded by a thick layer of hyaline cartilage; therefore, the elasticity and plasticity of the calcaneus is higher in young children compared with older children. Fractures of the calcaneus are seen more frequently in older children and adolescents. In contrast to adults, only

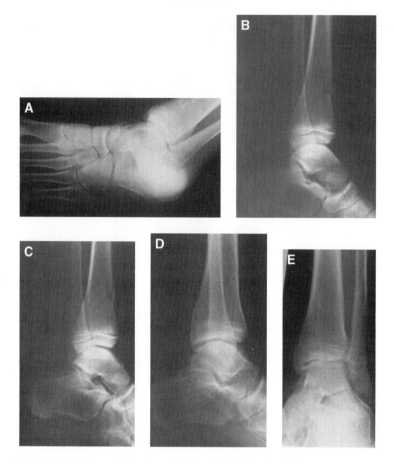

Fig. 9. Undisplaced fracture of the talar neck (*A*) and undisplaced shaft fracture of the distal tibia (*B*) sustained by a 15-year-old boy after colliding with a fence during tobogganing. (*C*) Image obtained before plaster cast application in plantiflexion. Correct alignment of the talar neck and anterior subtalar joint is visible. (*D, E*) At 18 months postinjury, a spontaneous arthrodesis of the anterior subtalar joint is evident. The posterior facet of the subtalar joint shows no signs of ankylosis. Clinically, there is pain and a mild posterior subtalar joint effusion (confirmed by MRI). An arthrodesis of the posterior part of the subtalar joint is planned.

a small number of calcaneal fractures in children are accompanied by spinal compression injuries [18]. Children also have fewer intra-articular fractures than adults, presumably because there is less exposure to trauma and any trauma that occurs is less severe [17]. In younger children, even simple falls can cause calcaneal fractures.

Fractures of the calcaneus can be classified according to Schmidt and Weiner [15] or according to Wiley's classification [18]. The latter divides calcaneal fractures into type 1 fractures, in which the fracture line does not involve the subtalar joint. These fractures include beak, vertical, horizontal, and avulsion fractures. Type 2 fractures involve the subtalar joint and are subclassified into undisplaced, tongue, displaced centrolateral, sustentaculum tali, and comminuted fractures.

All studies reporting larger series of calcaneal fractures in children mention difficulties and delay in diagnosis and the more benign nature of calcaneal fractures in children compared with adults [13]. The leading clinical sign of a calcaneal fracture is a painful calcaneus compression sign (pince-grip sign) and swelling of the heel. Radiographs in calcaneal fractures should consist of axial and lateral-medial images. The Böhler's angle (tuber joint angle) can be determined only by comparing radiographs of the uninjured calcaneus (Fig. 10) [19]. If available, MRI scans should be obtained in all calcaneal fractures. CT scans give the most accurate images in intra-articular fractures of the calcaneus and should be restricted to this type of fracture [20].

Careful soft tissue care is the major goal when managing calcaneal fractures. Therefore, initial treatment is directed toward the soft tissue, and repeated monitoring of the soft tissue situation is mandatory. Measurement of the foot compartment pressures should not be postponed when the trauma is severe or the swelling is progressing rapidly [21]. A primary compartment syndrome complicates displaced calcaneal fractures in children in up to 10% of cases. Missed foot compartment syndrome results in development of claw toes, foot nerve lesions, and severe foot deformities and growth disturbances [22].

Most calcaneal fractures in children can be treated by plaster cast application and non–weight bearing for 4 to 8 weeks. Undisplaced, stable, green stick–type extra-articular calcaneal fractures in young children consolidate within 3-4 weeks. Weight bearing should be delayed until pain has subsided. In contrast, fractures involving the articular surface of the subtalar joint (usually in older children) (Fig. 11) require immobilization and limitation of weight bearing up to 6 to 8 weeks. Even areas of avascular necrosis of the calcaneus usually heal within 2 to 3 months. Fractures of the calcaneus heal with an area of increased bone density, whereas the apposition of external callus is very limited. Non–weight bearing can be established by using crutches together with short leg casts or by the application of long leg casts with flexion of the knee or the application

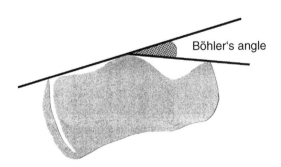

Böhler's angle

Fig. 10. Measurement of Böhler's angle for assessment of calcaneal fractures. Böhler's angle is compared in the injured and the noninjured contralateral calcaneus. Böhler's angle is usually about 30° (range, 17°–44°).

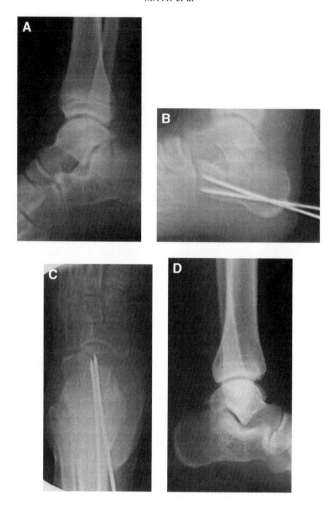

Fig. 11. (A) Minimally displaced fracture of the posterior subtalar joint facet of the calcaneus in a 12-year-old boy who was rolled over by a bus and who sustained multiple injuries. (B, C) Intra-operative image-intensifier views during percutaneous K-wire (diameter 2.0 mm) stabilization. (D) Four years postoperatively, there is no sign of deformation of the calcaneus, and the boy was walking without any difficulties.

of a patella tendon bearing together with an external lift on the bottom of the shoe for the uninjured leg. In cases with a significant flattening of Böhler's angle (Böhler's angle reduced by more than 10° in children 10 years or older or reduced more than 20° in children 6 to 9 years old compared with the normal contralateral calcaneus), the authors perform closed reduction and percutaneous pin stabiliza-tion through the heel apophysis. The authors insert canulated screws only in older children.

Open fractures of the calcaneus are mainly caused by lawn mowers or severe crushing forces. These injuries often require microsurgical repair using free-tissue transfer procedures to cover the soft tissue and bony defect. This process is accomplished using soft tissue flaps with or without additional bone grafts to restore the shape of the calcaneus. After initial debridement using pulse lavage management of the open injuries, the creation of an interdisciplinary treatment plan helps to cover the bone and soft tissue defects as soon as possible, limiting further tissue loss and minimizing the risk of subsequent infection.

Even in calcaneal fractures that have healed with a Böhler's angle less than that of the uninjured side, compensation by overgrowth of the inferior articular facet of the talus has been described in children [13]. Thus, the remodeling mechanism of the talus compensates for the depression of the calcaneal joint facet in an age-dependent manner. Therefore, most calcaneal fractures in children can be managed nonoperatively. Comminuted fractures of the calcaneus with significant depression of the subtalar joint area, however, should be reduced and stabilized by closed manipulation and K-wire or screw fixation through the heel or by open reduction internal fixation by way of a lateral L-shaped approach. In rare cases, comminution of the tuber area can result in a broadened and shortened heel, which in the authors' opinion, should be prevented by closed reduction and percutaneous insertion of two or three K-wires through the heel apophysis in the longitudinal axis of the calcaneus. This methodology helps to restore the tuber joint angle (see Fig. 10) and prevents varus malalignment of the posterior calcaneus after closed reduction.

Other avulsion fractures can occur in children. Isolated avulsion fractures of talocalcaneal ligaments (Fig. 12) in children are treated by below-knee plaster cast immobilization for 3 to 4 weeks and usually respond well to nonoperative management. Avulsion of the anterior process (joint facet edge) of the calcaneus sometimes results in a pain-free nonunion of the fracture (eg, fibrous union) [23]. In case of recurrent pain or swelling or recurrent trauma at the site of the nonunion, excision or screw fixation of the fragment may be considered, depending on the size and location of the fragment [24].

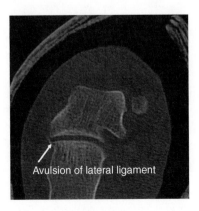

Avulsion of lateral ligament

Fig. 12. CT scan of an avulsion fracture of the lateral talocalcaneal ligament.

Fractures of the lesser tarsal bones

Fractures of the lesser tarsal bones (Fig. 13) occur as a result of massive deforming forces to the foot by direct trauma, by a fall from a height, or by a crushing mechanism [25]. Sometimes it is difficult to discern aseptic necrosis of the lesser tarsal bones from stress fractures or acute fractures. Due to the high forces involved in creating acute fractures of the lesser tarsal bones, strict monitoring and treatment of the soft tissue swelling within the first hours and days after trauma is strongly recommended. In the authors' opinion, the foot compartment pressures should not exceed 20 mm Hg (a limit of 30 mm Hg is recommended by Fulkerson and colleagues [26]). Treatment of fractures of the tarsal bones is generally nonoperative. Closed or open reduction using pin or screw fixation should be considered only when there are displaced fragments of adequate size. Multifragment fractures of the lesser tarsal bones are best treated by nonoperative means because open reduction of these injuries can jeopardize the remaining blood supply of the small fragments. These injuries are immobilized for 3 to 4 weeks using a below-knee plaster cast, and weight bearing is allowed after 1 to 3 weeks, depending on the remaining stability of the fracture.

Tarsometatarsal (Lisfranc's) injuries

The metatarsal bones and the tarsal bones are connected to each other by strong ligaments, with the weakest of these ligaments connecting the base of the first and second metatarsal bones. Therefore, tarsometatarsal dislocations are rare injuries in childhood [27,28]. The strongest ligaments keep the base of the second

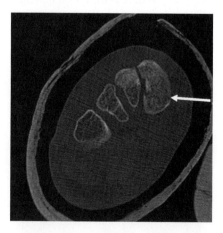

Fig. 13. Transverse CT scan of the lesser tarsal bones showing an undisplaced fracture of the first cuneiform. This 14-year-old boy was operating a motorcycle and was injured in a collision with a passenger car.

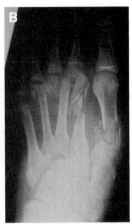

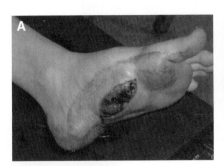

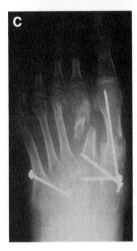

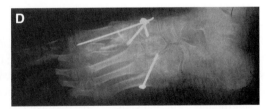

Fig. 14. (*A*) Open tarsometatarsal fracture dislocation (Lisfranc's joint dislocation) sustained by a 12-year-old girl when a horse stepped on her foot. Note the massive swelling. The compartment pressures measured in the foot compartments ranged from 50 to 65 mm Hg immediately after admission to hospital (primary compartment syndrome). (*B*) Fracture-dislocation of Lisfranc's joint and serial open metatarsal fractures. There are fractures of the first through fourth metatarsals, the first cuneiform, and the lateral part of the cuboid. Bases of the first through fourth metatarsals are dislocated to the peroneal side (Lisfranc's joint dislocation). (*C*) Following surgical decompression (fasciotomy) of foot compartments, the Lisfranc fracture dislocation was stabilized using canulated screws (diameter 3 mm) and one K-wire. (*D*) Radiograph taken 2 months postoperatively, before hardware removal and onset of free walking (hardware was removed because screws were crossing tarsal and tarsometatarsal joints and might have broken during unprotected weight bearing). There is a delayed union of the shaft fracture of the second metatarsal. The girl is able to walk without pain but has pain when participating in sports.

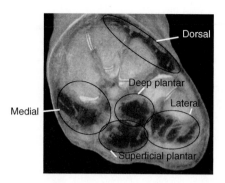

Fig. 15. Anatomic cross-section of the foot (cadaver specimen) at the region of the bases of the metatarsals close to the Lisfranc's joint; five compartments are marked (dorsal, medial, peroneal (lateral), superficial plantar, and deep plantar).

metatarsal in its position between the first and third cuneiform. All of the tarsometatarsal joints are in one plane, except for the second tarsometatarsal joint, which is located proximal to the other tarsometatarsal joints, thus providing a more stable position for the base of the second metatarsal [1].

Because very high forces are required to disrupt the Lisfranc's (tarsometatarsal) joint in a child, Lisfranc's injuries are at risk to be accompanied by a primary compartment syndrome (Fig. 14). Fasciotomy of all nine foot compartments (Figs. 15 and 16) using a medial, a lateral, and two parallel dorsal incisions for release of the interosseous midfoot compartments is done according to the same technique that is applied in adults.

Precise open reduction (preferably using a dorsal approach) of the joint dislocation around the base of the second metatarsal is key to achieving a good result [29]. After correct open reduction of the base of the second and first metatarsal and fixation by insertion of small canulated screws (diameter ~3 mm), the fourth and fifth metatarsals are stabilized using percutaneously inserted canulated screws (diameter ~3 mm) (see Fig. 14). Lisfranc's dislocations in children are sometimes accompanied by serial metatarsal fractures. In this

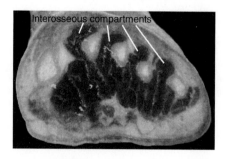

Fig. 16. Anatomic cross-section (cadaver specimen) at the level of the shafts of the metatarsals demonstrating the four interosseous compartments, which are marked, together with the five compartments described in Fig. 15.

situation, the authors stabilize the first and fifth metatarsal shafts and try to keep the heads of the second through fourth metatarsals in place by ligamentous traction. Using lateral and anteroposterior views, a Lisfranc's injury is sometimes difficult to detect. To determine the nature of a Lisfranc's injury exactly, a CT scan of the tarsometatarsal joint area is the most rewarding imaging option (Fig. 17). The most common radiographic sign on anteroposterior views is a widened gap (>3 mm) [13] between the first and second metatarsal base and between the first and second cuneiform (see Fig. 17A). Sometimes, small bone fragments are visible in the gap between the first and second cuneiform, indicating a bony avulsion of interosseous ligaments (see Fig. 17A).

For the postoperative period after screw fixation, the authors recommend application of a below-knee cast and non–weight bearing for 3 weeks and partial weight bearing for another 3 to 5 weeks. All joint-transfixing hardware should be removed before allowing full weight bearing without plaster cast immobilization. Some minimally displaced Lisfranc's injuries can be managed by closed

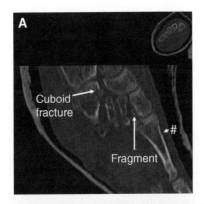

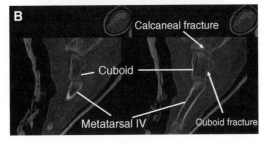

Fig. 17. (*A*) CT scan of a Lisfranc's fracture dislocation in a 14-year-old boy who collided with a passenger car while riding his motorcycle. Note avulsion of interosseous ligament together with a small bone fragment located between the first and second cuneiform together with widening of the gap between these tarsal bones. (*B*) CT scan of showing tarsometatarsal and calcaneotarsal dislocation together with angulation along the axis of the forth and fifth metatarsal. There is also an impacted compression fracture of the cuboid, a fracture at the base of the fifth and forth metatarsal, and an undisplaced fracture of the anterior edge of the calcaneus.

reduction and percutaneous K-wire (pin) fixation (if the reduction is unstable). K-wires can be left protruding through the skin [13].

In conclusion, key to the success of treatment in Lisfranc's injuries is the precise reduction and stabilization of the second metatarsal (most important), the first and fifth metatarsals, and the first and second cuneiform. In accordance with Wiley [28], the authors recommend long-term follow-up for Lisfranc's injuries in children.

Metatarsal fractures

Metatarsal fractures are frequent injuries in children, with the most vulnerable site of the metatarsals being the area of the neck. Fractures at the base of metatarsals can be accompanied by a tarsometatarsal dislocation. In case of serial fractures of metatarsals or following a crush injury, the foot must be carefully monitored for signs of compartment syndrome. Hypoaesthesia of toes, circumscribed paresthetic areas at the dorsal area of the first intermetatarsal space, bluish congestion of the toes, and massive swelling of the foot indicate compartment syndrome. To avoid development of claw toes and other serious foot deformities, a fasciotomy of all of the involved foot compartments must not be postponed.

Most solitary metatarsal fractures (Fig. 18A, B) in children are undisplaced and can be treated safely by using a molded, below-knee cast. Weight bearing can start as soon as the swelling and pain subside. The time of immobilization ranges from 3 to 4 weeks (see Fig. 18C, D). The most serious open metatarsal fractures are caused by lawn mowers [30]. Soft tissue care, adequate debridement, intravenous antimicrobial treatment, and minimal use of hardware are the cornerstones of treatment. When there is marked swelling of the foot together with displaced fractures of metatarsals, the reduction and percutaneous K-wire fixation of unstable fractures should be postponed until the swelling has somewhat subsided. Even in multiple metatarsal fractures, it is not necessary to stabilize all fractures. The most markedly displaced metatarsals and the metatarsals that outline the shape of the midfoot (first and fifth metatarsals) should be stabilized if indicated. K-wires from 0.8 mm to 1.4 mm in diameter are used for percutaneous fixation.

For closed manipulation, traction to the toes is applied and the K-wire is placed from the plantar aspect of the foot from distal to proximal. When open reduction is necessary, a dorsal incision is used to stabilize two metatarsals, and the K-wire (pin) is inserted into the fracture site under direct vision and drilled into the distal fragment until it exits through the plantar aspect of the forefoot. The fracture is reduced and the cut, proximal tip of the K-wire (pin) is guided into the medullary cavity of the proximal fragment. A split lower leg cast is applied, with sufficient space for the protruding tips of the K-wires (pins). K-wires are removed before the onset of weight bearing, approximately after 3 weeks. A nonunion of the metatarsals is rarely noted and treatment can be postponed unless

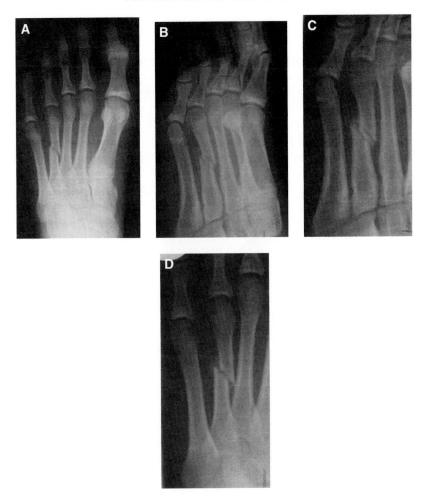

Fig. 18. (A, B) Minimally displaced fracture of the shaft of the fourth metatarsal in an 11-year-old girl who jumped from a balcony. (C, D) The patient was treated with a below-knee walking cast for 3 weeks. There is callus formation at the fracture site and no further displacement of the fracture (cf. panels A and B).

there is no involvement of the first or fifth metatarsal (outline of the foot) and no cross angulations, deformities, or discomfort (see Fig. 14C).

Comminuted fractures of the proximal part of the first metatarsal can occur in falls from a height ("bunk-bed injury") [31]. Avulsion fractures of the base of the fifth metatarsal are frequently observed in children active in sports [32]. The fracture line usually runs perpendicular to the axis of the fifth metatarsal. The fragment must not be confused with the secondary ossification center at the peroneal aspect of the base of the fifth metatarsal. Most fractures at the base of the fifth metatarsal can be treated successfully using a short leg cast for 3 to 4 weeks. When there is significant widening of the facture gap (width of gap

>8 mm), or in an active young athlete, screw fixation of the fragment is an option for treatment.

Stress fractures of metatarsals (most often, the shaft of the third metatarsal is injured) are observed in children active in running, soccer, or dancing, thereby representing an overuse injury. Stress fractures of metatarsals usually respond well to immobilization using a short leg walking cast for 2 to 3 weeks. It must be mentioned that the acute stress fracture of a metatarsal may not be visible on initial radiographs, and the apposition of callus or the decalcification of the fracture gap may not be visible on plain radiographs until 10 days after the fracture has occurred.

Fractures of phalanges

Fractures of the phalanges are frequently observed in children [33]. These fractures are usually caused by a direct kick of the toe to an object or by a forced angulation of the toe, most likely to the medial or lateral side. An osseous avulsion of the joint capsule and collateral ligaments in the great toe can cause a Salter-Harris type III injury. The osseous fragment is attached to the collateral ligament or joint capsule and can undergo significant rotation. Although fibrous healing can be achieved by nonoperative treatment, tenderness and swelling sometimes occur around the avulsed fragment, and even growth arrest of the physis has been described [1]. Therefore, the authors recommend open reduction and internal fixation of avulsed, rotated fragments of adequate size using K-wires of small diameter (<1 mm) or 1.3-mm titanium screws.

Mono- or bicondylar fractures are typical fractures of the head (trochlea) of the proximal phalanx of the great toe, and displaced fractures (fracture gap ≥2 mm, rotated fragments) should undergo open reduction and fixation as mentioned previously (Fig. 19). After operative management of toe fractures, the authors apply a short leg cast for 3 weeks. Phalangeal factures represent Salter-Harris type II epiphysiolysis or transverse shaft fractures. Closed reduction of a toe fracture using local or regional anesthesia and interdigital application of a handle of a pair of scissors or a pencil is sometimes required to correct gross angulations. Fractures of the lesser digits seldom require more than the application of tape. Taping is used to splint fractured toes to the adjacent, uninjured toes. Gauze or plastic foam padding is placed between the toes to prevent skin maceration. The tape is replaced every 5 to 7 days and the injured toe is checked for correct rotation. Children are advised to elevate the injured leg whenever possible and to wear wide shoes. Tapes are used for 3 weeks, and no further radiographic images are obtained in uncomplicated fractures.

In serial fractures of phalanges, the authors apply a below-knee plaster cast. In open fractures of toes, the authors close the wound, administer antibiotics for 3 to 5 days orally, and apply a below-knee cast. Fixation of unstable open toe fractures using K-wires (pins) of small diameter (<1 mm) is rarely necessary.

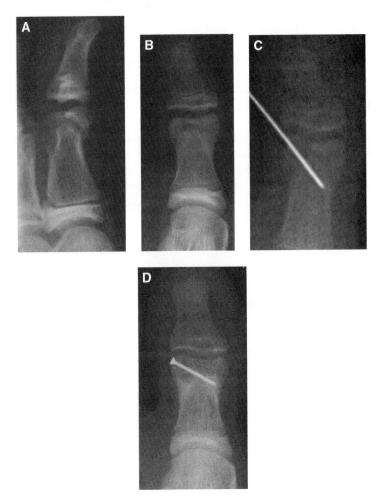

Fig. 19. (*A, B*) Displaced monocondylar fracture of the proximal phalanx (trochlea) of the great toe in a 10-year-old female gymnast who fell from monocycle during acrobatics. (*C*) After open reduction, the fracture was stabilized using one 1.3-mm titanium screw (intraoperative image-intensifier study). (*D*) At follow-up 6 months after injury, the girl was free of pain and actively participating in sports. The screw was not removed.

When children hit the tip of the great toe onto an object, epiphysiolysis of the distal phalanx can occur ("stubbed toe") [34,35]. This fracture easily becomes infected, and even osteitis can follow this innocent-appearing injury. Application of a below-knee plaster cast, elevation, limitation of weight bearing, and application of topical and orally administered antimicrobials are recommended together with evacuation of a subungual hematoma. The authors prefer fenestration of the proximal nail before reduction of the dislocated nail into its bed.

Dislocation of metatarsophalangeal or interphalangeal joints

Acute dislocations of toe joints require adequate reduction using local, regional, or general anesthesia. Traction is applied to the distal phalanx and, usually, reduction of the dislocated joint is achieved under image-intensifier control. After successful closed reduction, the injured toe is taped to an adjacent uninjured toe for 2 weeks.

In dislocations that are not recent and when there is interposition of soft tissues or sesamoid bones, open reduction has to be considered. The authors prefer a small dorsomedial or dorsolateral approach, and transfixation of the involved joint using K-wires (pins) of small diameter is sometimes necessary to prevent redislocation. The hardware is removed after 2 weeks and can be left protruding through the skin. After reduction, a short leg cast is applied for 3 weeks.

References

[1] Ogden JA. Skeletal injury in the child. 3rd edition. New York: Springer Verlag; 2000.
[2] Mulfinger GL, Trueta J. The blood supply to the talus. J Bone Joint Surg Br 1970;52:160–7.
[3] Jensen I, Wester JU, Rasmussen F, et al. Prognosis of fracture of the talus in children: 21 (7–34) year follow-up of 14 cases. Acta Orthop Scand 1994;65:398–400.
[4] Schuind F, Andrianne Y, Burney M, et al. Avascular necrosis after fracture or dislocation of the talus: risk factors, prevention. In: Arlet J, Ficat RP, Hungerford DS, editors. Bone circulation. Baltimore (MD): Williams and Wilkins; 1984. p. 393–7.
[5] Letts RM, Gibeault D. Fractures of the neck of the talus in children. Foot Ankle 1980;1:74–7.
[6] Marti R. Fractures of the talus and calcaneus. In: Weber BG, Brunner C, Freuler F, editors. Treatment of fractures in children and adolescents. New York: Springer; 1980. p. 376–87.
[7] Canale ST, Kelly Jr FB. Fractures of the neck of the talus. Long-term evaluation of 71 cases. J Bone Joint Surg Am 1978;60:143–56.
[8] Davy A. A propos de cas d'osteochondrite dissequante de l'enfant [Apropos the case of osteochondritis dissecans in the child]. Ann Chir 1961;15:311–6.
[9] Ly PN, Fallat LM. Transchondral fractures of the talus: a review of 64 surgical cases. J Foot Ankle Surg 1993;32:352–74.
[10] Yuan HA, Cady RB, DeRosa C. Osteochondritis dissecans of the talus associated with subchondral cysts. J Bone Joint Surg Am 1979;61:1249–51.
[11] Ferkel RD, Fasulo GJ. Arthroscopic treatment of ankle injuries. Orthop Clin North Am 1994; 25:17–32.
[12] Bryant DD, Siegel MG. Osteochondritis dissecans of the talus: a new technique for arthroscopic drilling. Arthroscopy 1993;9:238–41.
[13] Rockwood Jr CA, Wilkins KE, Beaty JH. Fractures in children. 4th edition. Philadelphia: Lippincott-Raven Publishers; 1996.
[14] Dimentberg R, Rosman M. Peritalar dislocations in children. J Pediatr Orthop 1993;13:89–93.
[15] Schmidt TL, Weiner DS. Calcaneal fractures in children. An evaluation of the nature of the injury in 56 children. Clin Orthop 1982;171:150–5.
[16] Linhart WE, Höllwarth ME. Frakturen des kindlichen Fußes [Fractures of the child's foot]. Orthopade 1985;15:242–50.
[17] Schanz K, Rasmussen F. Calcaneus fracture in the child. Acta Orthop Scand 1987;58:507–9.
[18] Wiley JJ, Profitt A. Fractures of the os calcis in children. Clin Orthop 1984;188:131–8.
[19] Böhler L. Die Technik der Knochenbruchbehandlung [The treatment of fractures]. 12./13. Auflage. Wien: Maudrich; 1963.

[20] Rosenberg ZS, Feldman F, Singson RD. Intra-articular calcaneal fractures: computed tomographic analysis. Skeletal Radiol 1987;16:105–13.

[21] Mittlmeier TM, Mächler G, Lob G, et al. Compartment syndrome of the foot after intraarticular calcaneal fracture. Clin Orthop 1991;269:241–8.

[22] Myerson M, Manoli A. Compartment syndromes of the foot after calcaneal fractures. Clin Orthop 1993;290:142–50.

[23] Gellman M. Fracture of the anterior process of the calcaneus. J Bone Joint Surg Am 1951;33: 382–6.

[24] Degan TJ, Morrey BF, Braun DP. Surgical excision for anterior-process fractures of the calcaneus. J Bone Joint Surg Am 1982;64:519–24.

[25] Hunter LY. Stress fractures of the tarsal navicular bone. Am J Sports Med 1981;9:217–9.

[26] Fulkerson E, Razi A, Tejwani N. Review: acute compartment syndrome of the foot. Foot Ankle Int 2003;24:180–7.

[27] Mantas JP, Burks RT. Lisfranc injuries in the athlete. Clin Sports Med 1994;13:719–30.

[28] Wiley JJ. Tarso-metatarsal joint injuries in children. J Pediatr Orthop 1981;1:255–60.

[29] Myerson M. Tarsometatarsal joint injury: subtle signs hold the key. Physician Sports Med 1993; 21:97–107.

[30] Shereff MJ. Complex fractures of the metatarsals. Orthopedics 1990;13:875–82.

[31] Mayr J, Seebacher U, Lawrenz K, et al. Bunk beds—a still underestimated risk for accidents in childhood? Eur J Pediatr 2000;159:440–3.

[32] Dameron TB. Fractures and anatomical variations of the proximal portion of the fifth metatarsal. J Bone Joint Surg Am 1975;57:788–92.

[33] Buch BD, Myerson MS. Salter-Harris type IV epiphyseal fracture of the proximal phalanx of the great toe: a case report. Foot Ankle 1995;16:216–9.

[34] Jahss MH. Stubbing injuries to the hallux. Foot Ankle 1981;1:327–32.

[35] Pinckney LE, Currarino G, Kennedy LA. The stubbed great toe: a cause of occult compound fracture and infection. Pediatr Radiol 1981;138:375–7.

ELSEVIER
SAUNDERS

Clin Podiatr Med Surg
23 (2006) 191–207

CLINICS IN
PODIATRIC
MEDICINE AND
SURGERY

Preconditioning Principles for Preventing Sports Injuries in Adolescents and Children

Mark D. Dollard, DPM[a,b,c,*], David Pontell, DPM[c,d,e], Robert Hallivis, DPM[c,d,e]

[a]*Private Practice, Loudoun Foot and Ankle Center, Suite 111, 46440 Benedict Drive, Sterling, VA 20164, USA*
[b]*Department of Orthopedics, Georgetown University Medical Center, Washington, DC, USA*
[c]*Podiatric Surgical Residency Program, Inova Fairfax Hospital, Fairfax, VA, USA*
[d]*Department of Podiatric Medicine, Temple University School of Podiatric Medicine, USA*
[e]*Private Practice, Dominion Foot and Ankle Consultants PC, Suite 101, 3301 Woodburn Road, Annandale, VA 22003, USA*

In the United States, more than 30 million children and teenagers are expected to participate in all levels of sports and recreational activities. Even with the best coaching and training facilities, 3% to 11% of these children between the ages of 5 and 15 years old become injured. National statistics provided by the National Safe Kids Campaign and the American Academy of Pediatrics have disclosed that 3.5 million injuries each year occur within this 5- to 14-year-old age group. Hospital emergency rooms may expect up to 775,000 injuries to children in this age group. This age group comprises roughly 40% of all emergency room visits for sports-related injuries. The two major injury groups include acute traumatic injuries and overuse injury syndromes. The demands of individual, team, and recreational sports may account for the different injury occurrences within each group. Although the prevalence of injuries in organized sports tends to dominate in the age group from 9 to 14 years old, in younger age groups, both playground entry level and bicycle injuries usually account for the remainder. The practitioner providing medical service to any organized sports program should be aware of the percentage of athletes injured within specific sports and the specific types of injuries unique to the sport (Fig. 1). Typically, the following percentages

---

* Corresponding author. Loudoun Foot and Ankle Center, Suite 111, 46440 Benedict Drive, Sterling, VA 20164.
E-mail address: mdollard@erols.com (M.D. Dollard).

0891-8422/06/$ – see front matter © 2006 Elsevier Inc. All rights reserved.
doi:10.1016/j.cpm.2005.10.003
podiatric.theclinics.com

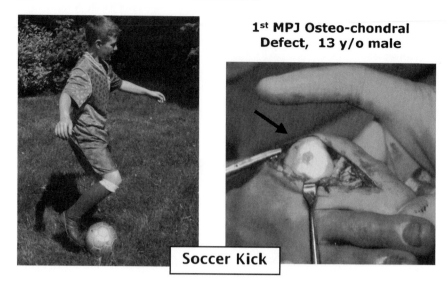

Fig. 1. Specific sports injuries. (Courtesy of M.D. Dollard, DPM, Sterling, VA.)

of players are injured in these specific sports: (1) basketball, 15%; (2) football, 20%; (3) soccer, 22%; (4) baseball, 25%; and (5) softball, 12%. As the demand for greater competitive performance filters down into the younger age groups, prolonged practice routines are now accounting for almost 50% of all overuse injuries encountered in the middle- and high-school years [1]. Sixty percent of all injuries incurred in organized sports-related activities often occur from organized practice sessions. It is the goal of this article to present principles of pre-conditioning and injury prevention.

Injury prevention

The causes of sports-related injuries is related to the physiologic age of the youth athlete rather than to chronologic age [2]. The dynamics of any sport place extraordinary demands on individual tissue systems that are dependent on the status of the epiphysis, bone structure, and general growth status [3]. Not all tissue systems are at equal risk for damage. In the case of soft tissue muscle-tendon injuries, most follow two general patterns: injuries to muscle-tendon units crossing two joints and injuries to muscle-tendons units that decelerate joints by excessive tension from eccentric muscle contractions [4] Most commonly, muscles whose origin and insertion cross two joints are most vulnerable to injury [2]. Typical examples in this group are the Hamstrings and Achilles tendons. Because these muscles span two joints, they may experience extensive tensile elongation, producing tears in their fibers. The next most vulnerable muscle groups tend to be those muscles that experience an eccentric contraction to decelerate motion at a joint. An eccentric contraction is one in which muscle tension increases in a muscle as it contracts to resist a force that attempts to overstretch the muscle's length. A common example of an eccentric stretch would be the increasing tension in the biceps muscles of the arm holding a steady position at the elbow while a hand weight is gradually lowered onto a table. The quadriceps tendon is another eccentric muscle unit that provides eccentric resistance while preventing hyperflexion of the knee at heel strike in runners. Another eccentric example is the anterior extensor muscles of the tibia. These muscles slow the dropping of the forefoot at heel strike in a gradual manner through an eccentric contraction. Overuse of these extensor muscle units creates susceptibility to periosteal tears at their origin, creating "shin splints."

Injury prevention starts with identifying the causes and factors of poorly conditioned athletes. Such factors include improper training techniques, environmental hazards, physiologic weakness, and nutritional status. This article focuses on improper training techniques and cites where intensity, duration, and training frequency can induce pathologic problems in the lower extremity. The basic concepts in preseason conditioning and the vocabulary that sports medicine specialists must know to converse intelligently with coaches, trainers, and strength conditioners are emphasized.

Preseason screening: Tanner Body Index

A child's physiologic age is predominantly more important than his or her chronologic age in assessing individual ability to acclimate functionally to a specific youth sport. The Tanner Body Index is a method of classifying the youth athlete according to his or her physiologic development with pubescent maturation [5]. The Index has four classifications: stages I, II, III, and IV. For boys, maturation is based on the growth of pubic hair and genitalia. For girls, staging is based on breast formation. Early prepubescent Tanner stages I and II are characterized by pretestosterone level increases and immaturity in the musculoskeletal system. Youths in this stage are best assigned to nonimpact sports, such as running. Tanner stages III (midpubescent) and IV (postpubescent) are characterized by periods of growth and skeletal maturation. At the midpubescent stage III (boys aged 12–15 year, girls aged 10–13 years), it is precisely these growth spurts that make the child most vulnerable to injury in two basic ways: joint tightness with limiting ranges of motion and peak epiphyseal vulnerability. Growth spurts may create asymmetry of long bones and an imbalance in opposing muscle-tendon units. The subchondral bone and physis become easily susceptible to microtrauma [3]. Associated muscles and tendons must stretch out to meet these new bone lengths. The muscles become functionally short while accommodating to new bony anatomic lengths. This tightness limits the effective range of motion about their respective joints. As an example, Achilles tendon equinus is often the precursor to calcaneal apophysitis and pronation syndromes in the foot. During this time, flexibility programs must be instituted to regain lost range of motion about these tightened joint structures.

Tanner stage III prepubescent youths (aged 11–13 years) are experiencing a period of peak gain in height. Such growth spurts produce stress points at the expanding physis at its weakest time. Impact sports are most apt to induce disturbances with growth plates at this stage [6]. Such concern should be monitored in Tanner stage III youths.

Regardless of the extent of preseason physical examinations and body indexing, three basic areas of functional skills evaluation are important. Three most useful functional tests are; the Functional Rhomberg Test for postural balance and pelvic strength integrity, the 150% Body Strength Rule for general muscle strength, and the Agility Index for neuromuscular reactivity [7].

Functional Rhomberg Test

This test evaluates the athlete's ability to handle weight loads about the axial skeleton during sport activity to maintain balance. The Functional Rhomberg Test specifically evaluates the ability of muscles about the pelvic girdle to stabilize balance. The athlete is asked to stand and balance upright over a single limb. In performing this drill, the athlete should be able to stand upright and one legged on the supporting limb. This position is held for 30 seconds without tilting or angling the upper torso over the support leg for balance. Alternately, on command, the youth athlete should be able to stand up onto his or her toes 10 times without excessively shifting his or her body position or losing balance. Any tendency for the athlete to sway or swagger over the support limb raises suspicion regarding inadequate strength to stabilize the pelvis (Fig. 2). Pelvic girdle

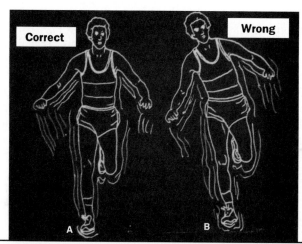

The athlete should be able to stand upright on the supporting limb, one legged, for 30 seconds without tilting his body position for balance; or on command stand up onto his tip toes 10 times without shifting body position

Fig. 2. Functional Rhomberg Test. (Courtesy of M.D. Dollard, DPM, Sterling, VA.)

muscular strength is essential to maintain proper axial posture and stability for avoidance of spinal and lower extremity pathologic injury. Preseason programs should be designed to strengthen the hip flexors and extensors, the lateral stabilizers, the abdominal muscles, and the hamstring muscles about the pelvic girdle to ensure axial pelvic stability (Fig. 3).

150% Body Strength Rule

Because sports loads may amplify body weight strain onto the axial skeleton between 2.5 and 4 times normal body weight, an athlete must be able to squat press at minimum of 150% of his or her body weight before participating in any type of ballistic activity, such as explosive jumping sports or fitness aerobics. Tests to evaluate such strength levels may include squat presses of weights at loads of 150% of the athlete's body weight with free-weight or squat-press machines. Not until the athlete is able to readily squat press 150% of his or her body weight should the youth be allowed to participate in competitive sports (Fig. 4).

Agility Index for neuromuscular reflex reaction

Many sports entail a competitor's agility to react, twist the torso, shift position laterally, and execute contorted movements. Agility testing is essential in

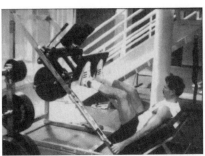
Hip Flexors/Extensors

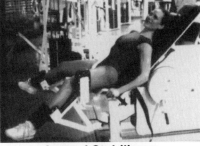
Lateral Stabilizers

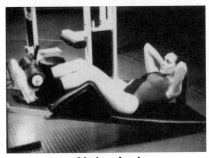
Abdominals

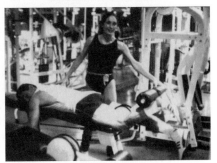
Hamstrings

Fig. 3. Strengthening the pelvic girdle muscle. (Courtesy of M.D. Dollard, DPM, Sterling, VA.)

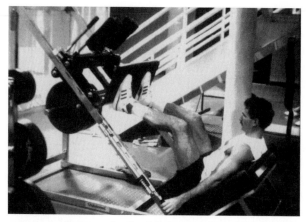

- **Since sports may induce a load > 2.5x body weight, then an Athlete or Fitness participant must be able to squat press 150% of their body weight before participating in any type of ballistic activity such as Aerobics or Explosive Sports**

Fig. 4. Minimum body strength rule. (Courtesy of M.D. Dollard, DPM, Sterling, VA.)

evaluating neuromuscular reflex reactivity in the athlete. The Agility Index drill is designed by placing several construction cones aligned in a zigzag pattern stretched across a 30-yd distance. The athlete is then asked to run and cut in and around the cones in a figure-of-eight weaving pattern within a specific period of time while performing specific agility maneuvers at each station along the way (Fig. 5). Any evidence of stumbling or difficulty in executing these maneuvers

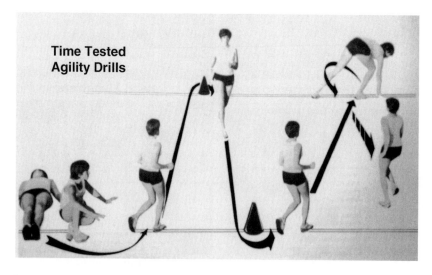

Fig. 5. Agility Index. (*Adapted from* Kuland D, editor. The injured athlete. Philadelphia, JB Lippincott; 1982. p.107; with permission.)

should raise suspicion of immaturity in neuromuscular agility. The athlete may need to undergo specialized agility skills training before being placed in competitive sports events.

Designing preconditioning programs

Acclimatization: preconditioning

Clinicians need to be aware of the concept of acclimatization as it relates to preconditioning programs. In a more basic sense, acclimatization understands that a body that has been relatively inactive for a period of time needs to adapt to a new level of exercise intensity, duration, and frequency. There are four basic concepts involved in the design of a preconditioning program: strength training, flexibility training, agility training, and performance training. Peak performance training routines are designed to accelerate the body's cyclic ability to cope with the rigors of sports by peaking midseason to prevent the body from experiencing general fatigue and body system failure. Performance training areas are discussed first.

Preconditioning for performance

Performance training
Performance has a mixed definition depending on the motivations of the athletes and their supporters. Goals can vary from physical achievement in skills performance to win-loss records in youth sports. Regardless, the clinician should be aware that performance in training circles is often broken down into three areas: sports-specific skills, technique execution, and cyclic peaking.

Sports-specific skills. Individual sports naturally have greater demands on specific muscle groups. The football quarterback designs a training routine emphasizing the upper torso for throwing. The track and field hurdler is more apt to concentrate on lower extremity development. It is beyond the scope of this article to outline the training routine of each specific sport. For those interested, however, we would highly recommend becoming involved with such organizations as the National Strength and Conditioning Association, National Athletic Trainers Association, and American College of Sports Medicine and their publications, which report on specific sports, as well as their training routines to achieve peak performance. These programs outline preseason and off-season weight training and conditioning drills. These individual training programs target the various muscle groups that are specific to athletic function in sport.

Sports technique execution: improper technique, asymmetry, and repetition.
Improper technique. Valuable information is gained by monitoring the technical execution of various training routines in sport. Clinicians are often con-

fronted with the long distance runner who displays improper technique with excessive twisting pelvic sway or extended knee strike. Poor running techniques can induce problems such as piriformis sciatic nerve entrapment syndrome in which the sciatic nerve is sandwiched between the pyriformis and gemellus muscles in the pelvic region, causing radiating pain (paresthesias) into the leg [8].

Asymmetric routines.   Few coaches are aware of the potential consequences of asymmetry in their designed training regimens. A commonplace example is with competitive weightlifting, in which a "clean and jerk maneuver" explosively lifts heavy barbell weights over weightlifter's head [9]. This maneuver is often performed with one leg repetitively thrusting forward and the other leg thrusting backward for balance. By failing to alternate both legs to ensure symmetric training, individual muscle groups become overtrained. These overtrained muscle groups overpower their antagonist. We have seen severe functional scoliosis develop in weightlifters as a result. A practitioner must be aware of any asymmetry involved in the athlete's training routine to best judge how and why injuries are occurring that may differ from one limb to the another. In another example, soccer players experience a different set of injuries in their planted foot as opposed to their kicking foot. Soccer preseason drills need to challenge both limbs equally.

Repetitious maneuvers.   Repetitive motion creates fatigue stress. Ballet maneuvers represent such repetitive motion injuries. The repetitive extremes of inversion and eversion rolling of the foot, known as "sickling," raises the body up to the point position on the toes. This action constantly jams the os trigonum bones behind the ankle and fatigues the flexor hallucis longus tendons. Fibrous polyp formation or tears in the flexor hallucis longus may plague the ballet dancer. Differentiating between a fracture of the os trigonum versus polyps within the flexor hallucis longus is often difficult even with sophisticated diagnostic tests, such as MRI [10–12].

Performance peaking: Cyclic periodization and supercompensation

A major goal of this review is to provide the clinician with an understanding of the principles of cyclic training to enhance peak performance throughout the athletic season. Periodization is best defined as a system for applied cyclic variances in training intensity and workload throughout the competitive season to acclimate the athlete's body to reach higher levels of performance in avoidance of fatigue or injury [13,14]. This step-graded approach supercompensates the athlete to achieve higher levels of performance and endurance [15]. In general, the Cyclic 3:1 Day Rule is instituted by trainers and coaches to accomplish this cyclic task. Simply explained, athletic training is progressively intensified over 3 days and then followed immediately by a mandatory 1 day of rest. In general, exercise physiologists profess that protein synthesis needed for recovery occurs not during exercise periods but during rest periods. Exercise periods break down protein tissue. Rest periods are absolutely necessary for protein tissue recovery [16].

Micropeaking

Micropeaking is defined as a period of four daily practice sessions in which the athlete's body is gradually stressed to higher levels of performance in three of the four sessions. The fourth session becomes a vital period of rest. After the rest session is completed, a new cycle of training starts. The body is now physiologically able to adapt and accommodate to higher workloads placed on it by super-compensating to a higher level of performance (Fig. 6). At the critical start point of a new four-session cycle, a new progressively higher load or intensity is placed on the body. Because recovery is allowed during the preceding rest period, the body is able to rebound to a higher level of stress management. Typically, in a 1-week scenario, as workloads are progressively increased to an established stress set point, the body fatigues by the end of the third day. Determining that set point is discussed in a later section. For now, programs for strength and weight training establish the set point as a measure matched against a weight index, the *One Repetition Max (1RM)*. The 1RM refers to the maximum weight that a person can lift for a total of 10 repetitions, reaching a "max-out" fatigue point. The initial 1RM is set before any starting point in a cyclic training program. After the rest session, a new 1RM is then reset to a progressively higher maximum weight level for the next cycle of weight training [17]. This graded training principle is called *progressive resistance exercise* (PRE). Alternately, if the goal is to increase endurance levels, the 10% Endurance Rule applies. This set point is indexed by

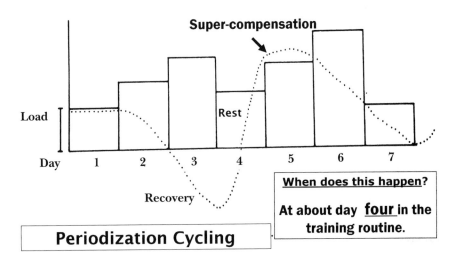

Fig. 6. Supercompensation. (*Adapted from* McFarlane B. Dynamics of adaptation: supercompensation. NSCA Journal 1985;7(3):44–5, with permission.)

no greater than a 10% increase in duration and intensity of exercise over any week's time [18].

Macropeaking

Macropeaking is best defined as a monthly cycle of several week-long sessions graduated over the course of the entire season, peaking the athlete three quarters of the way through the season to maximize his performance. The Cyclic 3:1 Day Rule applies here as well. Taking the same rule as with 1 week of microloads and applying the rule to the 4 weeks on a monthly scale, athletes may be able to avoid common overuse injuries. By the fourth month of the competitive season, general body fatigue may begin to overshadow performance. With macropeaking principles, workout sessions tend to increase in their intensity and load over 3 weeks of workouts followed by 1 week of low-level activity for rest and rebound (Fig. 7). Otherwise, it is well known that overuse injuries appear at roughly the third week after initiating a poorly developed noncyclic sports training program. At this point, the body is at its most vulnerable point from fatigue strain on skeletal bone remodeling. Many participants in recreational or fitness activities, such as aerobic dance or organized sports, often break down physically at this 3-week point by failing to adhere to these cyclic principles of training. Our experience with high incidences of injuries 3 weeks into a typical health club aerobic dance program testifies to the high occurrence of metatarsal stress fractures, tibial stress fractures, and other overuse injuries at this point.

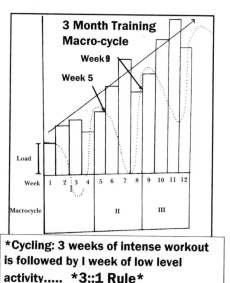

Fig. 7. Performance peaking. (*Adapted from* McFarlane B. Dynamics of adaptation: supercompensation. NSCA Journal 1985;7(3):44–5, with permission.)

Therefore, cyclic training best requires a mandatory session of rest after three sessions of activity on a weekly, monthly, and season-long schedule.

Preconditioning for flexibility, agility, and strength

Flexibility training

As discussed previously, physiologic hazards associated with prepubescent Tanner stage III youth are caused by sudden tendon tightness about joints induced by long bone growth spurts. Flexibility programs are essential at this youth level. Adapting the body's response to enhance the myotatic reflex and Golgi tendon organ (GTO) systems within muscle and tendon is vital to flexibility standards. The myotatic reflex response invokes an intramuscular contraction to avoid tearing from overstretching. The GTO systems are a complex of intermuscular reflexes that balance relaxation of antagonist muscle groups with the agonist muscle. This allows the agonist muscle to move a joint through its full range of motion unimpeded. This concept is referred to as reciprocal inhibition. Without precise coordination of these two muscle reflexes, shock absorption at joints is compromised. Athletic performances are hindered, and bone fracture syndromes are induced. Three different types of techniques are available to improve flexibility: static and passive stretches, proprioceptive neuromuscular facilitation (PNF) buddy stretches, and ballistic-bouncing stretches [19]. Immediately before any stretching drill, an athlete should warm up his muscle groups with a prestretch brisk walk or light jog.

Static stretch techniques are the preferred method to increase flexibility in youth groups. An individual muscle is passively stretched by the athlete to a maximum length for 30 seconds, which is repeated for three to five sets. These stretch drills are easily understandable, readily demonstrable, and easily reproducible by the youth athlete. The key muscle groups for general body stretching should include the lumbar torso, the Achilles tendons, the hamstrings tendons, the lateral hip iliotibial band tendons, and the iliopsoas muscle group (Fig. 8). Youth athletes at Tanner stages I, II, and III respond well to static stretch techniques.

Proprioceptive neuromuscular fascilitation (PNF) stretches involve a buddy system in which a counterforce is placed against a contracting muscle to invoke reciprocal relaxation in its antagonist muscle [20]. A counterforce is held by a buddy for 6 seconds against the desired agonist muscle (eg, hamstring) while that muscle is voluntarily contracted. This eventually fatigues the myotatic reflex. The muscle contraction is then relaxed, and the buddy passively stretches the fatigued agonist muscle-tendon unit while the antagonist muscle (eg, quadriceps) is voluntarily contracted for 3 seconds to invoke a GTO response by the antagonist, which reciprocally causes relaxation in the stretched agonist, the hamstring. A far greater outstretch of the agonist hamstring can be executed (Fig. 9). The athlete must have a well-developed nervous system to take advantage of this PNF technique. Because of the complexity in the execution of PNF techniques, they are usually reserved for mature Tanner stage IV athletes.

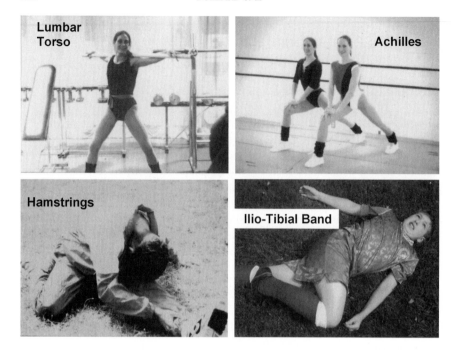

Fig. 8. Static stretches. (Courtesy of M.D. Dollard, DPM, Sterling, VA.)

Ballistic stretches are an extraordinarily delicate series of controlled bouncing drills that rapidly invoke myotatic and GTO function with functional agility [19]. Because of their powerful effect, requiring accurate balance, they are reserved for use in supervised elite ballistic sport programs, such as volleyball, basketball, or sprinting. These active agility stretches are often used within preparatory drills known as plyometric reaction drills for sports requiring explosive power. In a more basic form, these plyometric agility drills can be modified to a less intense degree for use in a precondition program to awaken senescent muscles, increase neuromuscular recruitment, and enhance reflex reactivity.

Agility training: plyometric ballistic exercise preconditioning

Plyometric training is a controlled system for converting kinetic energy into explosive power by fine-tuning coordination between myotatic and GTO reflex systems, thus enhancing the body's dynamic proprioceptive abilities. This is accomplished through a series of jumping drills. The basic drill in plyometric conditioning uses rebounding jumps into a series of agility drills (Fig. 10) [4,16,21]. Great explosive power is produced when the neuromuscular proprioception reflexes are challenged by experiencing a controlled sudden eccentric stretch followed by a rebounding concentric contraction. Our clinic has designed a plyometric circuit training system based on stations positioned around a running track (Fig. 11) [22]. At each circuit station along the track, the athlete is

Hamstring contracted for 6 seconds against partner upward resistance	Quad contracted for 3 seconds while partner stretches the Hamstring

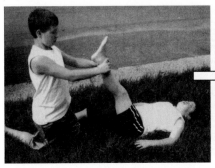 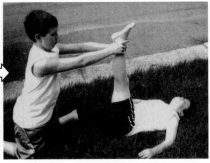

Hamstring muscle's Golgi tendon organ causes the Quadriceps muscle to relax	Quadriceps muscle's Golgi Tendon organ causes the Hamstring to relax

Fig. 9. PNF stretches. (Courtesy of M.D. Dollard, DPM, Sterling, VA.)

expected to perform any of a series of the following drills within a hopscotch grid: running in-place, jump rope, chopping drills, carioca scissoring, single leg jumps, double leg jumps, hopscotch forward, hopscotch zigzags, and double hops. Depending on the athlete's Tanner stage, low-level weights may be added progressively to overload the muscles and supercompensate the athlete to higher performance levels (Fig. 12).

Strength training preconditioning

Basic principles of weight training
    The *progressive overload principle* holds that a muscle must be progressively challenged with a greater resistance or load to improve strength or endurance.

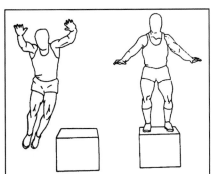 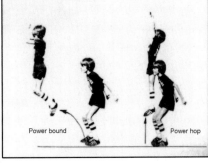

Fig. 10. Dynamic agility drills. (*Adapted from* Kuland D, editor. The injured athlete. Philadelphia: JB Lippincott; 1982. p. 141; with permission.)

"Dollard Hopscotch Circuit System"
Dollard 1984

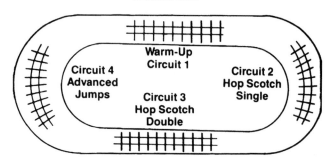

Fig. 11. Plyometric agility training. (*Adapted from* Dollard M. Plyometric ballistic conditioning. Aerobics and Fitness 1985:34; with permission.)

Strength training assists the body in maintaining postural integrity (endurance) or work output performance (strength). Muscle physiology, fiber typing, or the aerobic and/or anaerobic demands of an individual sport dictate training approaches with weights [23,24].

Explosive power sports usually call on fast-twitch type IIb muscle fibers, which function for high work force for a short duration of activity. These fiber types have great tension potential but are anaerobically inefficient in energy consumption. Training these muscles usually focuses on strength principles aimed at quickly lifting heavy weights through three sets with a low number of

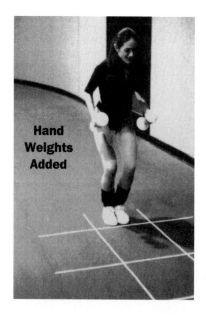
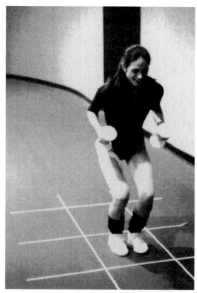

Fig. 12. Plyometrics with weights. (Courtesy of M.D. Dollard, DPM, Sterling, VA.)

repetitions (eg, <9 repetitions). Endurance sports, such as cross country, typically call on slow-twitch type I fibers with activity of long duration with high aerobic efficiency. Training these muscles focuses on endurance principles aimed at lifting low weights through three sets with a high number of repetitions (eg, >15 repetitions). General maintenance with weight training often must combine endurance and strength principles, because postural muscles of balance in the pelvis and spine tend to be "endurance"-oriented slow-twitch fibers responsible for holding axial balance position over long periods of time. Performance muscles of power in the extremities tend to be "strength"-oriented fast-twitch fibers responsible for quick forceful actions.

Whether for strength or endurance training, the standard index for the amount of weight used as a training tool is based on the *one repetition maximum* (1RM) set point. Now that the 1RM is understood, the typical weightlifting schedule for endurance or strength training is designed over the course of sessions according to the 3:1 rule. Weight loads are gradually increased until muscular contractions fatigue at the *max-out* point for any particular set of muscles. The following schedule is typical:

> *Strength muscle training (type II fibers [eg, quadriceps]):* weight at 80% to 100% 1RM (three sets with 8–9 repetitions)
>
> *Endurance muscle training (type I fibers [eg, abdominals]):* weight at 60% 1RM (three to four sets with 15 repetitions)

Successful weight training seeks to challenge a muscle's tension potential throughout its entire fiber length and its full range of motion. Weight training through concentric contractions (ie, shortening tension) or eccentric contractions (ie, lengthening tension) may differ depending on the actual equipment in use. This specific discussion is beyond the scope of this article. Interested readers may seek further information on the tension-curve relationship brought about by weight training equipment using various resistance techniques: (1) isometric resistance (ie, same length with increased tension), (2) isotonic variable resistance (ie, same tension with variable resistance [eg, Nautilus with free weights]), or (3) isokinetic resistance (ie, variable speed with variable resistance [eg, Cybex with machines]).

Weight training and children

Weight training in children is a controversial issue. An inadequate testosterone level is often cited as the reason why weightlifting for strength gain has little value for fitness or athletic conditioning in prepubescent children [25] Some views hold that children cannot benefit from any form of weight training until they achieve Tanner stage III. Sewall and Micheli [26] studied weight training in children in Tanner stages I and II, reporting significant gains in muscular strength in response to progressive muscle training. Heija found that high-school athletes participating in a comprehensive weight training program had approximately one third fewer injuries. The American Orthopedic Society for

Sports Medicine has recommended that weight training for prepubescent children follow these guidelines: (1) no maximal 1RM lifting, (2) limit weight training to two to three times a week at 20 to 30 minutes each session, and (3) no more than three sets of lifting with six to nine repetitions per set. In prepubescent Tanner stage II children, technique training is best emphasized over strength training to improve neuromuscular development and recruitment. In later Tanner stages III and IV (usually in children aged 14–17 years), the principles of progressive resistance exercise can be acceptably individualized per athlete and specific sport needs.

Summary

Preseason preconditioning can be accomplished well over a 4-week period with a mandatory period of rest as we have discussed. Athletic participation must be guided by a gradual increase of skills performance in the child assessed after a responsible preconditioning program applying physiologic parameters as outlined. Clearly, designing a preconditioning program is a dynamic process when accounting for all the variables in training discussed so far. Despite the physiologic demands of sport and training, we still need to acknowledge the psychologic maturity and welfare of the child so as to ensure that the sport environment is a wholesome and emotionally rewarding experience.

References

[1] Requa RK. The scope of the problem: the impact of sports related injuries. Proceedings of Sports Injuries in Youth, Surveillance Strategies. Bethesda (MD): National Institute of Arthritis and Musculoskeletal and Skin Diseases. National Institutes of Health; Bethesda, MD. p. 19.

[2] Malina RN. Adolescent changes, size, build, composition and performance. Hum Biol 1974;46: 117–49.

[3] Hackney RG. ABC of sports medicine, nature, prevention and management of injury in sport. BMJ 1994;308:1350–9.

[4] Lundin P. A review of plyometric training. National Strength and Conditioning Association Journal 1985;7(3):69–74.

[5] Tanner JM. Growth at adolescence. 2nd edition. Oxford (UK): Blackwell Scientific; 1962.

[6] Carty H. Children's sports injuries. Eur J Radiol 1998;26(2):163–76.

[7] Kulund D. The injured athlete. Philadelphia: JB Lippincott; 1982.

[8] D'Ambrosia R, Drez Jr D. Prevention and treatment of running injuries. New Jersey: Charles B Slack; 1982.

[9] Takano B. Coaching optimal technique in the snatch and the clean and jerk. National Strength and Conditioning Association Journal 1987;9(6):52–6.

[10] Soloman R, Micheli L. Concepts in the prevention of dance injuries. In: Shell CG, editor. The dancer as athlete. Champaign, Illinois: Human Kinetics; 1984. p. 201–12.

[11] Hardaker W, Erickson L, Myers M. Foot and ankle injuries in dance and athletic. In: Shell CG, editor. The dancer as athlete. Champaign, Illinois: Human Kinetics; 1984. p. 31–41.

[12] Khan K, Brown J, Way S, et al. Overuse injuries in classical ballet. Sports Med 1995;19(5): 341–57.

[13] Charniga A, Gambetta V, Kraemer W, et al. Periodization. Roundtable discussion. National Strength and Conditioning Association Journal 1986;8(5):12–22.

[14] Pedemonte J. Foundations of training periodization. National Strength and Conditioning Association Journal 1986;8(3):62–6.

[15] McFarlane B. Supercompensation. National Strength and Conditioning Association Journal 1985;7(3):44–6.

[16] Bielk E, Chu D, Costello F. Practical considerations for utilizing plyometrics. National Strength and Conditioning Association Journal 1986;8(3):14–22.

[17] James S. Periodization of weight training for women's gymnastics. National Strength and Conditioning Association Journal 1987;9(1):28–32.

[18] O'Neill D. Preventing injuries in young athletes. Journal of Musculoskeletal Medicine 1989;11:21–35.

[19] Knortz K, et al. Flexibility techniques. National Strength and Conditioning Association Journal 1985;7(2):50–3.

[20] Jacobson B. Neuromuscular facilitation, the long term plateau effect. National Strength and Conditioning Association Journal 1986;8(6):62–6.

[21] Chu D. Plyometric exercise. National Strength and Conditioning Association Journal 1984:56–7.

[22] Dollard M. Plyometric ballistic conditioning, a system for pre-conditioning the aerobic exerciser. Aerobics and Fitness 1985;3(2):33–5.

[23] Shibinski M. The adolescent athlete, teaching and coaching young athletes in the weight room. National Strength and Conditioning Association Journal 1985;7(4):60–2.

[24] Beckham-Burnett S, Grana W. Safe and effective weight training for fitness and sport [abstract]. Journal of Musculoskeletal Medicine 1987;4(11):26–46.

[25] Webb DR. Strength training in children and adolescents. Pediatr Clin North Am 1990;37: 1187–210.

[26] Sewall L, Micheli LJ. Strength training for children [abstract]. J Pediatr Orthop 1986;2:143–6.

ELSEVIER
SAUNDERS

Clin Podiatr Med Surg
23 (2006) 209–231

CLINICS IN
PODIATRIC
MEDICINE AND
SURGERY

Sports Injuries in the Pediatric and Adolescent Foot and Ankle: Common Overuse and Acute Presentations

David Pontell, DPM[a,b,c,*], Robert Hallivis, DPM[a,b,c], Mark D. Dollard, DPM[c,d,e]

[a]Department of Podiatric Medicine, Temple University School of Podiatric Medicine, 8th at Race Streets, Philadelphia, PA 19107, USA
[b]Private Practice, Dominion Foot and Ankle Consultants PC, Suite 101, 3301 Woodburn Road, Annandale, VA 22003, USA
[c]Podiatric Surgical Residency Program, Inova Fairfax Hospital, Fairfax, VA, USA
[d]Private Practice, Loudoun Foot and Ankle Center, Suite 111, 46440 Benedict Drive, Sterling, VA 20164, USA
[e]Department of Orthopedics, Georgetown University Medical Center, Washington, DC, USA

Care of the youth athlete requires detailed knowledge of developmental anatomy and injuries or syndromes that present with significant frequency in a given sport. A basic approach to the history and physical examination is presented, followed by specific syndromes and conditions encountered, both of which are related to overuse and acute injury. We conclude with a discussion of factors to be considered when assessing youth athletes and their readiness to return to play.

History and physical examination in pediatric foot and ankle sports injuries

Eliciting a thorough history relating to the chief complaint is essential to making an accurate diagnosis. Such practice facilitates ranking of differential diagnoses and aids, for example, in distinguishing between an acute injury and overuse syndromes. This is of particular significance in the skeletally immature

* Corresponding author. Dominion Foot and Ankle Consultants PC, Suite 101, 3301 Woodburn Road, Annandale, VA 22003.
  E-mail address: dpontell@cox.net (D. Pontell).

0891-8422/06/$ – see front matter © 2006 Elsevier Inc. All rights reserved.
doi:10.1016/j.cpm.2005.10.005 *podiatric.theclinics.com*

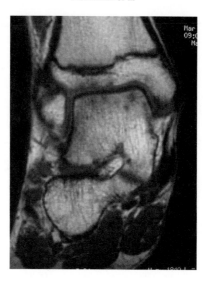

Fig. 1. A 12-year-old boy with insidious onset of rearfoot and lateral "ankle" pain. MRI confirms talocalcaneal middle facet coalition and a nondisplaced medial osteochondral lesion of the talar body.

patient in whom congenital and/or developmental disorders, such as tarsal coalition and the osteochondroses, are so prevalent (Fig. 1). Likewise, an accurate history tends to focus the physical examination on areas of greatest concern. This being said, evaluation of the child or adolescent athlete should always include consideration of past medical history and review of systems so that nontraumatic (or posttraumatic) etiologies are considered. Examples would include septic arthritis, reflex sympathetic dystrophy syndrome/chronic regional pain syndrome (RSDS/CRPS), or neoplasia (benign and malignant), whose initial presentation may be preceded by or mimic an acute (otherwise trivial) or overuse injury

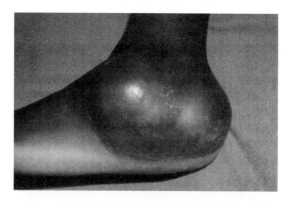

Fig. 2. A 12-year-old boy who presented with gross irregularity of soft tissue contour in the lateral ankle of 3 months' duration, which was initially mistaken for an ankle sprain. An open biopsy confirmed soft tissue sarcoma requiring amputation.

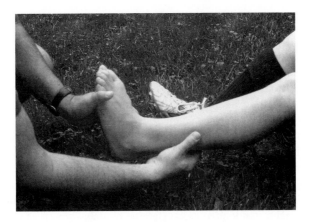

Fig. 3. Range of motion, muscle tone and guarding, and joint stability are tested in a non–weight-bearing attitude (open kinetic chain) before assessment of weight-bearing mechanics. Note is made of edema, ecchymosis, and deformity.

(Fig. 2). Illustrative of this concept is the study of Wilder and colleagues [1], who describe their experience with 70 pediatric subjects treated for RSDS, 50% of whom had identified discrete injuries preceding their symptoms incurred in an organized sport. Physical examination of the pediatric or adolescent athlete with a foot or ankle injury must include evaluation in the open kinetic chain to assess range and quality of joint motion as well as manual muscle testing (Fig. 3). Guarding secondary to pain and muscle bulk and tone are assessed at the same time. Areas of palpable tenderness, swelling, and ecchymosis are noted. Likewise, skeletal deformity and abnormalities of soft tissue contour are noted.

Station and gait are assessed to the extent possible, given the nature and degree of injury, with attention to the axial and appendicular skeleton. Position and function in the cardinal body planes should be noted. Particular attention is paid to the structure and mechanics of the spine and to the functional limb length, talocalcaneonavicular complex, ankle joint, flexor and extensor function, and digits at the metatarsophalangeal joint (MTPJ) level. Once this initial evaluation is complete, plain radiographs are ordered (if indicated) and assessed. Laboratory and more advanced imaging studies are obtained as indicated.

Overuse injuries of the foot and ankle in pediatric and adolescent athletes

Overuse injury has been defined by Herring and Nilson [2] as resulting from "repetitive application of submaximal stress to otherwise normal tissues, overwhelming the normal repair process." Recent decades have seen increasing numbers of skeletally immature athletes competing in such sports as gymnastics, diving, and figure skating, putting these younger athletes at risk for these types of injuries. Several authors have pointed to changing patterns and frequency of injuries in skeletally immature athletes, which seems to be coincident with younger and younger players participating in their respective sports [3,4]. Competitive youth athletes may find it necessary to participate in rigorous training programs, although overuse injuries are by no means limited to elite athletes. Recreational youth and "travel" teams may require four or more practice sessions per week, for example, in such sports as soccer, football, swimming, and ice hockey. With the evolution of "single-sport" youth athletes, the potential for year-round, overuse of particular muscle-tendon units and sports-specific skeletal structures is increased. Likewise, the polysport athlete may also be at risk. Such adolescents may compete in soccer, lacrosse, and baseball on a given weekend, allowing inadequate time for recovery of stressed soft tissue and bony structures.

Micheli [4] has identified that overuse injuries about the foot and ankle may present in a tendon (tendonitis), bone (fatigue or stress type fracture), or tendon insertion (apophysitis) or in cartilage (articular, epiphyseal plate, or apophysis). In fact, these are common presenting complaints in practices that treat skeletally immature athletes.

Osteochondroses

Once believed to be a group of conditions whose primary etiology was local arterial insufficiency leading to frank osteonecrosis, it is now appreciated that this is a heterogeneous group of disorders whose etiologies range from normal variants of ossification (Sever's phenomenon) through ischemic necrosis secondary to a discrete traumatic event (Kohler's disease) [5].

Calcaneal apophysitis

Calcaneal apophysitis is among the most common presenting diseases in foot and ankle practices that see youth athletes and, in our experience, the most common cause of heel pain in the growing athlete. Although Sever [6] is generally credited with the original description of this disorder, no reference to osteochondrosis is made. The disease typically presents in 10- to 13-year-old children (male predominance) and is frequently bilateral but often asymmetric relative to symptom level [7]. There is frequent association with tight Achilles tendons and a recent growth spurt. Most authors point to an association with pes planovalgus, but our experience suggests that youth athletes with cavus foot types are also at risk secondary to functional pseudoequinus and the position and prominence of the calcaneal apophysis.

Findings may vary from mild palpable pain about the heel circumference to calcaneal compression tenderness (virtually pathognomonic), which may be so severe as to make weight bearing intolerable. A clear history of a recent increase in training or competition is often elicited. Sports that require a high percentage of running and jumping, such as soccer, basketball, track, and gymnastics, are commonly associated [7]. Plain radiographs may be normal, but multipartite apophyses with or without sclerosis are common (Fig. 4). Alterations, such as

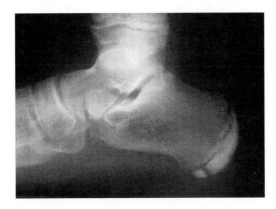

Fig. 4. A 12-year-old male soccer player with calcaneal apophysitis treated with rest, a short-leg ambulatory splint, and custom foot orthoses.

periosteal new bone or bony destruction, rule out this disorder, and further imaging should be performed to define these "look-alike" conditions (eg, stress fracture versus neoplasm).

Micheli [7] has reported a retrospective follow-up on a group of 85 patients treated for this disorder. All patients received supervised physical therapy (gastrocnemius-soleus stretching), and most (75%) received a "heel wedge," heel cup, or Plastizote foot orthoses. In this study, the removable inserts were used in athletic and conventional shoes, barefoot gait was prohibited, and nonsteroidal anti-inflammatory drugs (NSAIDs) were not used. All patients improved, and return to activity was well documented in 50 patients at an average of 2 months (mean of 2.2 months in male patients and mean of 1.6 months in female patients, range: 1–6 months) [7]. Two patients were reported to have recurrent heel pain at 1 year after initial onset; both were successfully treated with a regimen similar to the original, which returned them to their desired activities [7].

Our practice experience suggests that initial treatment must include discontinuation of running and jumping activity until symptoms abate. Likewise, supportive strappings, heel cups, and intermittent icing can be helpful for symptom reduction. Finally, short-leg cast immobilization for 2 to 4 weeks remains the "gold standard" in cases refractory to less restrictive measures or in patients for whom relative rest (in the context of their daily lives) is difficult to achieve. We have also used ambulatory short-leg splints as long as compliance can be reasonably ensured.

The osteochondritis associated with the tarsal navicular (Kohler's disease) presents with tenderness in the medial arch that may be severe enough to produce a limp. This is recognized to occur more frequently in boys than in girls (6:1 ratio), may be bilateral, and presents with a peak incidence in children aged 2 to 9 years [8]. A history of trauma may or may not be appreciated.

Radiographs are revealing for sclerosis and apparent fragmentation and narrowing of the ossification center of the involved side. It should be noted that

30% of boys and 20% of girls that are asymptomatic demonstrate irregular ossification of the navicular [9]. When clinical diagnosis and plain films are inadequate, nuclear medicine scanning or MRI may be helpful in ruling out significant avascular necrosis (AVN) [8,10]. Cessation of running and jumping activities should be instituted, whereas cast immobilization for 6 to 12 weeks may facilitate early return to activity [11].

Apophysitis associated with the growth center at the base of the fifth metatarsal (Iselin's disease) is a relatively common overuse injury in the pediatric athlete involved in running sports. It presents with point tenderness with or without swelling directly over the lateral base of the fifth metatarsal. Schwartz and colleagues [12] suggest that metatarsus adductus may be a risk factor for this condition secondary to malposition of the fifth metatarsal base. Although no history of acute injury is often elicited, occasional reporting of a supination type injury may be noted. It has been suggested that this overuse injury may be underreported or mistaken for a fracture (Fig. 5). Simons and Sloan [13] pointed out that the apophyseal plate does not extend into the fifth metatarsal–cuboid joint or to the interval between the fourth and fifth metatarsals, helping to distinguish true fractures from this condition. Rest and discontinuation of the exacerbating activity, foot strapping with or without aperture padding over the tuberosity, ice, and immobilization are the mainstays of treatment. Physical therapy, including proprioception training with a tilt board, may be helpful in avoiding repetitive supination mechanism type reinjury. Athletes may return to play when they are comfortable enough to play without favoring the area that would have previously elicited pain and avoidance.

Stress fractures

The incidence of stress fractures in youth athletes is believed to be increasing with year-round sports participation [10]. The most common areas for stress

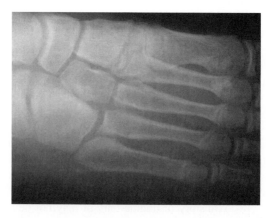

Fig. 5. A 14-year-old skateboarder with a nondisplaced distal fifth metatarsal shaft fracture. His initial diagnosis was a fifth metatarsal base fracture (this is an asymptomatic apophysis).

fractures in children are the tibia, fibula, pars interarticularis, and femur [14]. Proximal first, second, and third metatarsal stress fractures are reported in pediatric dancers [15]. Although these are seen with less frequency than in adults, this stress type injury should be suspected in any weight-bearing bone that presents with point tenderness and no history of discrete acute injury. This is inclusive of "irregular" bones, such as the cuneiforms, cuboid, and hallux sesamoids, all of which are at risk for fatigue type fracture. Three-phase technetium bone scanning is especially useful when the history and physical examination point to this diagnosis in the face of negative plain radiographs.

Special mention should be made regarding female athletes in whom amenorrhea is recognized. The association of amenorrhea with eating disorders and osteoporosis is well documented [16]. A complete history and physical examination, along with appropriate laboratory testing and subspecialty referral, should be undertaken in addition to treatment of the skeletal injury.

Among the most important diagnostic imperatives for those caring for young athletes is recognition of navicular stress fracture. Bennell and Brukner [17] have documented the incidence of navicular stress fractures compiled from 18 large studies as comprising anywhere from 0% to 28.6% of injuries in one study of track and field athletes. Overuse, combined with reduced vascularity of the central one third of the navicular, is hypothesized to contribute to the etiology of this injury. Foot type has not been demonstrated to be associated with a relative risk, although equinus contracture may be a contributing factor [18]. The history often reveals the insidious onset of pain located over the medial or dorsal midfoot, which is exacerbated by activity and relieved by rest. It is likely that this partial recovery, along with reduced clinical suspicion, is responsible for regular reports of delayed diagnosis, often months in duration. Physical examination is revealing for palpable tenderness over the "N" spot (dorsal, central navicular) [18]. Plain radiographs may be entirely normal, whereas technetium scanning

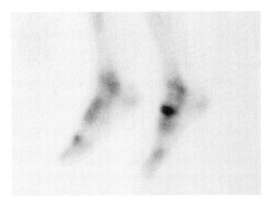

Fig. 6. A 16-year-old female basketball and soccer player with pain in the left medial arch of 4 months' duration, who was unable to continue playing. A technetium bone scan confirms a navicular stress fracture and rules out AVN. Percutaneous fixation and 3 months of rehabilitation allowed her return to play without sequelae.

reveals intense increased uptake in the entire navicular (Fig. 6). CT scanning may help to distinguish between nondisplaced incomplete injuries and displaced fractures (vertically oriented), which may guide management decision making.

Although nonsurgical care often suffices (non–weight-bearing cast mobilization for 6 weeks or longer), there is a significant incidence of delayed or nonunion. Percutaneous screw fixation and open reduction internal fixation (ORIF) with autogenous grafting may be necessary for resolution. Patients and their families must be counseled on the high degree of patience necessary to tolerate the slow recovery that characterizes this injury. The average time of return to activity has been reported to be 5.6 months [18].

Acute foot and ankle injuries in the youth athlete: classification of epiphyseal injuries

The history of our understanding of epiphyseal injuries is a long and fascinating one, dating from the writings of Hippocrates. It was not until John Poland wrote a classic paper on the subject in 1898 that these injuries were clearly understood. In 1963, Salter and Harris [19] published an outstanding summary of the pathophysiology, recognition, treatment, and classification of these injuries. It is this latter classification that has the most current application.

The Salter-Harris classification consists of five types of injury [19]. Type I is a line of cleavage confined to the physis without involvement of the metaphysis or epiphyseal ossification center (Fig. 7). This type accounts for 6% to 8.5% of all injuries and occurs most commonly in the phalanges. Type II is by far the most common, accounting for 73% to 75% of all epiphyseal injuries. The line of fracture is through the physis and then extends through a margin of the metaphysis, separating a variably sized triangular metaphyseal fragment referred to as the "corner sign." The distal radius accounts for one third to one half of the injuries in this category. The distal tibia, distal fibula, and phalanges account for most of the remainder. Type III injuries account for 6.5% to 8% of all epiphyseal injuries. The fracture runs vertically or obliquely through the epiphysis and then extends horizontally to the periphery of the physis, separating a portion of the epiphysis. Normally, displacement is minimal. There is no associated fracture of the metaphysis. The injury is usually encountered at the distal tibia or distal phalanx. The injury often occurs after there is partial closure as a result of normal maturation of the physis.

Type IV is a vertically oriented splitting compression force that extends across the epiphysis, physis, and adjacent metaphysis, separating a portion consisting of the metaphysis and the epiphysis. This accounts for 10% to 12% of all epiphyseal injuries. The most common sites are the lateral condyle of the humerus and the distal tibia. Type V injuries are rare, accounting for less than 1% of all injuries. This type of injury is associated with no immediate radiologic findings. It is presumed to be attributable to a pure crushing injury of the epiphysis or the

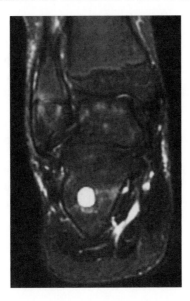

Fig. 7. A 14-year-old tennis player with an acute lateral ankle injury. Point tenderness over the lateral malleolus and focal marrow edema on both sides of the distal fibular physis confirm the diagnosis of a Salter-Harris type I fracture. An incidental finding of a calcaneal cyst is noted.

physis, resulting in damage to the perichondral ring, and occurs most commonly at the knee [19].

Anatomy of the epiphysis

The epiphysis, at the end of a long bone, is the site where cartilage is converted into bone and where growth in length occurs. The normal epiphyseal plate, located between the epiphysis and the metaphysis of a long bone, is composed of four distinct layers: (1) the germinal zone, or resting cells adjacent to the epiphyseal ossification center, consists of small cells; (2) the proliferating zone, a zone of flattened cells arranged in columns; (3) the hypertrophic zone, comprised of swollen vacuolated cells maintaining the columnar arrangement; and (4) the zone of provisional calcification at the metaphysis. The physis is encircled by the perichondral ring, a layer of fibrocartilaginous tissue contiguous with the adjacent periosteum of the metaphysis and epiphysis.

The bony surface of metaphyses and epiphyses is irregular or corrugated and consists of small bony projections, undulations, knobs, and ridges termed *mammillary processes*. These features stabilize the adhesion between the physis and adjacent bony surfaces but may also serve to concentrate stresses, leading to crack failure, and thereby determine the site and direction of epiphyseal injury.

With regard to the arterial blood supply, fortunately, at most sites, the metaphysis and epiphysis receive their supply from distinctly separate sources, such that a line of fracture through the growth plate does not interfere with the arterial supply of the epiphysis or the metaphysis. The metaphysis is supplied at its center by branches of the nutrient artery and at its periphery by numerous small branches of the periosteal arteries originating from the diaphysis. The vascular supply of the epiphysis consists of several periosteal vessels that arise on larger arteries about the joint. With this dual arrangement, the epiphyseal arteries supply nourishment for cartilaginous growth, whereas the metaphyseal arteries nourish ossification. Vascular complications to an epiphysis after injury are thus unusual.

Salter and Harris [19] have postulated that the fracture takes place at the weakest part of the epiphysis, which is located at the level of the hypertrophying cells. More recent experimental studies in animals have shown that the position of the fracture line is, in fact, variable and may sometimes include portions of the other three zones.

Acute ankle injuries

Fractures of the distal tibial and fibular physes constitute 4% of all ankle injuries [20]. The most obvious difference between fractures in children or adolescents versus adults is the presence of an epiphysis. The distal tibial and fibula growth plates form a plane of weakness, resulting in injury patterns markedly different from those seen in adults. Ligaments in the skeletally immature child may be stronger than the physis, increasing the risk of physeal injury over that of ligamentous sprain [20,21].

An important aspect that must be considered in pediatric injuries about the ankle is the closure of the distal tibial epiphysis. Closure of the distal tibial epiphyseal plate proceeds in two directions. The initial one is a near-central fusion site, which is then followed by fusion of the posteromedial and antero-lateral growth plate segments. This process occurs over an 18-month period anytime between the ages of 10 and 18 years and plays an integral role in the mechanism of injury of triplane and Tillaux ankle fractures [22].

Specific classifications and mechanisms of epiphyseal ankle injuries have been studied on an extensive basis. Dias and Tachdjian [23] have devised a clear and comprehensive classification system using Lauge-Hansen guidelines, foot position, and direction of force, which also correlates with the Salter-Harris classification [19].

The classification system devised by Dias and Tachdjian [23] involves four mechanisms: supination-inversion (grade 1: Salter-Harris types I and II, grade 2: Salter-Harris types III and IV), supination-plantarflexion (grade 1: Salter-Harris type II), supination–external rotation (grade 1: Salter-Harris type II), and pronation-eversion-external rotation (grade 1: Salter-Harris type II). In each of the mechanisms, the first term represents the fixed position of the foot at the time of injury and the second term represents the direction of abnormal force being transmitted to the ankle joint. Each mechanism has a correlation with the epiphyseal injury classification of Salter and Harris [19].

Under the classification system of Dias and Tachdjian [23], however, two other patterns of ankle fractures seen in children are not included. The first is a Salter-Harris type III injury of the distal tibial epiphysis, first described by Klieger and colleagues [24]. The other is the triplane fracture.

Landin and Danielsson [25] extended the classification system proposed by Dias and Tachdjian [23]. In their classification system, they included groups with a more adult fracture pattern. The fracture groups 1 through 7 are the same as those described by Dias and Tachdjian [23]. Group 8 is a Tillaux fracture, which is a Salter-Harris type III lesion of the anterolateral part of the distal tibial epiphysis (see Fig 7; Fig. 8). It is generally produced by a supination–outward rotation force. Group 9 is a triplane fracture, which is a Salter-Harris type II through IV fracture, with fracture lines in all three planes. The fracture lines are caused by a combination of plantarflexion and outward rotation. Group 10 and 11 are avulsion fractures from the lateral malleolus and medial malleolus, respectively. Groups 12 and 13 consist of cases with epiphyseal lines partially or completely closed and fractures with an appearance usually seen among adults. Group 14 is made up of combinations of fractures with an adult appearance. Group 15 are fractures that do not fit within the other subtypes included in the present classification system [25].

Salter-Harris type I and II fractures of the distal fibula are among the most common fractures seen in the athletic child (see Fig. 7) [26]. Supination and external rotation; pronation, eversion, and external rotation; and supination and

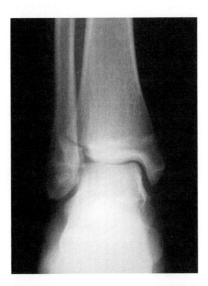

Fig. 8. A 14-year-old boy with a Tillaux fracture sustained during Tae Kwon Do training. The CT examination (see Fig. 9) confirmed 5 mm of displacement, which required percutaneous reduction and fixation.

plantarflexion can cause varying degrees of ankle ligamentous and bony injury, resulting in a Salter-Harris type I or II fracture pattern of the distal fibula and tibia. It is a supination-inversion mechanism that usually causes a Salter Harris type III or IV fracture of the distal tibia and has a greater chance for growth arrest [27].

The most common acute injury of the foot and ankle is the Salter-Harris type I fracture of the distal fibula. This is the childhood equivalent of a lateral ankle sprain in the skeletally mature patient. This fracture usually occurs after an inversion injury. Radiographs are typically normal, and the diagnosis is made by careful physical examination. Palpation demonstrates tenderness localized to the physis of the lateral malleolus. Treatment is a short-leg walking cast for 3 to 4 weeks. Rarely, there are growth arrests associated with this injury. In those cases in which the fractures are displaced, the families should be educated about possible epiphyseal arrest and subsequent ankle valgus development [28].

Salter Harris type II fractures of the distal tibia are also common. With this fracture, however, there is a significant incidence of epiphyseal arrest within this area [29]. Closed reduction may be difficult to maintain and may require internal fixation with percutaneously placed Kirschner wires. The fibula often fractures also, but most fibular fracture can be treated with simple closed reduction [28].

The most common Salter-Harris type III fracture is a Tillaux fracture of the distal lateral tibia (see Fig. 8; Fig 9). This is an isolated fracture of the lateral portion of the distal tibial physis that occurs with external rotation [20]. Such fractures occur in teenagers who are close to skeletal maturity of the distal tibia epiphysis. As the medial portion of the distal tibial physis closes at the end of adolescence, external rotation athletic injuries may result in a fracture of the anterolateral quadrant of the tibial physis. The pull of the anterior tibiofibular

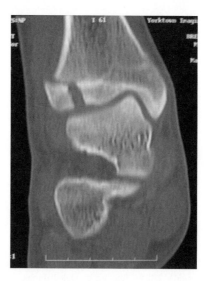

Fig. 9. Coronal CT image of a 14-year-old boy with a displaced Tillaux fracture incurred during Tae Kwon Do training, which required reduction and fixation.

ligaments results in avulsion of the anterolateral aspect of the distal tibial epiphysis. In the child, avulsion of the epiphysis is limited to the anterolateral part, because epiphyseal fusion has occurred at the medial and posterior areas of the distal tibial epiphysis. The fused parts of the plate are no longer the weak points but are of increased structural strength, which accounts for the pattern of fracture. This results in a Salter-Harris type III injury [26]. This fracture can be seen on plain radiographs of the ankle. The distinguishing features of the fracture are a vertical line extending from the ankle joint in the central to lateral area of the distal tibia superior into the epiphyseal plate and then extending laterally. The lateral film often shows the avulsed fragment displaced anteriorly. If the displacement is small, the fracture may only be evidenced by a slight widening of the growth plate laterally [28]. Many of these fractures are nondisplaced or minimally displaced and can be treated in a long-leg cast for 6 weeks. If there is displacement greater than 2 mm, open reduction and internal fixation should be performed. Options for fixation include smooth Kirschner wires or cortical screws [20,26,27].

Another type of epiphyseal injury is the so-called "triplane" ankle fracture. This fracture is defined as one in which the fracture plane has sagittal, transverse, and coronal components [30]. It consists of a vertical fracture of the epiphysis, a horizontal cleavage plane within the physis, and an oblique fracture of the adjacent metaphysis. Triplane fractures account for approximately 6% of all distal tibial epiphyseal injuries. Because of the increasing number of variants and the way this fracture presents on plain radiographs, it is often a confusing injury to diagnose accurately.

Two-, three-, and four-part triplane ankle fractures have been described in the literature [30–37]. Triplane fractures are caused primarily by shearing and avulsion forces. Specifically, the forces reputed to produce triplane fractures are isolated external rotation of the foot at the ankle, isolated plantarflexion of the foot, or a combination of both mechanisms [32,38,39]. Pure external rotation has support as the major force, because internal rotation of the foot (reversal of the insult of force) reduces the fracture at surgery.

Cooperman and coworkers [30] believed that the exact anatomy of the triplane fracture depends not only on the forces involved at the time of injury but on the stage of fusion of the epiphyseal plate in its different parts. A maturing partially fused epiphysis probably is a prerequisite for the occurrence of this fracture. Depending on the maturation sequence of the physis, a variable pattern can appear in the fracture, which is most evident in the variations in size of the metaphyseal fragments and location of the sagittal fracture lines.

This injury must be suspected in any child who shows evidence of injury near the end of the tibia. The child is unwilling to bear weight on the leg or limps. There is local tenderness and swelling at the epiphyseal plate. If there is significant injury at the plate, there is malalignment of the joint as well. Accurate diagnosis of an epiphyseal injury depends on obtaining radiographs in at least two planes. Comparison views of the contralateral limb may be necessary to define the injury accurately [40].

A thorough examination of plain anteroposterior and lateral radiographs enables one to make the diagnosis. A Salter-Harris type III fracture is visualized on the anteroposterior film, with the lateral view demonstrating a Salter-Harris type II or IV fracture. The location of the sagittal fracture through the epiphysis, as seen on an anteroposterior radiograph, can vary from medial to lateral. It may constitute up to 40% to 50% of the width of the epiphysis, with a range of displacement of 1 to 4 mm [38]. The percentage of metaphysis that is included in the posterior triangular spike as well as the length of this fragment can also vary greatly. It has been described to vary in height from 1 to 4 mm, with 0 to 4 mm of posterior displacement [38]. Additionally, a fibula fracture may or may not be noted. If present, it usually occurs 4 to 6 cm proximal to the tip of the lateral malleolus and runs obliquely from posterosuperior to anteroinferior. Whenever this combination of radiographic findings is encountered in the adolescent patient, the only possible explanation is a triplane fracture.

Although the diagnosis of a triplane fracture can be made from radiographs, the exact configuration of the fracture may be of greater difficulty to determine unless a great deal of distraction exists at the fracture site; therefore, advanced diagnostic tests must be obtained.

Although polytomography was once suggested as the best means of classifying triplane fractures, the CT scan has replaced it as the best modality to evaluate this complex fracture. CT can be used to evaluate and classify injuries already established on the basis of plain radiographs more fully. With CT, it is much easier to delineate the configuration and the degree of distraction of the fracture fragments. In fact, it has been recommended that CT scans be taken in all cases of triplane ankle fractures that have undergone closed reduction and show adequate reduction on plain films. This should ensure that adequate reduction of all fragments in all planes has truly been obtained [41].

If CT scans show a successful closed reduction, a conservative approach is advisable. The long-term prognosis should be good after 4 to 6 weeks of above-the-knee cast immobilization. This is followed by 4 weeks of below-the-knee cast immobilization, allowing partial weight bearing. Gradual return to activity is then encouraged, and physical therapy is instituted [42].

One reported barrier to closed reduction is an associated fibular fracture, whether a greenstick fracture or a complete fracture occurred. Because the ligament attachments between the fibula and the lateral part of the epiphysis are strong, the fibula remains attached to the lateral epiphysis regardless of the amount of displacement between the tibial components of a triplane fracture. Consequently, any fibular deformity can be expected to make closed reduction of a triplane fracture difficult [30].

Most authors agree that a two or three-fragment fracture displaying 2 mm or more of displacement on plain radiographs after closed reduction has been attempted needs to proceed to open reduction and internal fixation. In cases in which closed reduction fails or in which more than 2 mm of displacement still exists, open reduction and internal fixation are required. As with other fractures involving open growth plates, fixation must be aimed at providing anatomic reduction and rigid internal fixation without placing compressive devices across the epiphysis.

The configuration of the posterior metaphyseal spike and attached portion of the epiphysis lends itself to reduction with cancellous or cortical bone screws, using the lag screw technique. When possible, two screws should be used to allow superior fixation and earlier rehabilitation. Often, fixating this fragment moves the anterior fragments into place. Therefore, no attempt at reduction of the anterior fragments should be made until the posterior metaphyseal spike is anatomically reduced. In cases of two-fragment fractures, no additional fixation may be required. In cases of three-fragment fractures, the separate anterior fragment must also be reduced accurately and rigidly fixated to resist postoperative distraction and complications later on. Preferred methods of fixation include smooth or threaded pins driven from a medial to lateral direction across the epiphysis. Smooth pins may also be placed across the physis if necessary, but plans for their removal should be made before healing. Postoperative care is similar to that of a patient who has undergone closed reduction. Because of rigid internal fixation, however, range-of-motion exercises may be instituted earlier, which necessitates the use of a removable below-the-knee air cast after the 4 to 6 weeks of above-the-knee cast immobilization [42].

Complications of epiphyseal ankle fractures

Fractures that cross the epiphyseal plate with displacement of the fragment can lead to premature closure of the epiphyseal plate and deformity of the leg. Salter and Harris [19] have shown experimentally that accurate reduction and internal fixation may prevent growth deformity, and it is known that accurate reduction is also essential for a smooth joint surface. Accurate reduction and internal reduction should be considered in children with epiphyseal fractures involving the articular surface that do not allow accurate reduction by closed methods. With triplane fractures, however, these two complications are rarely seen clinically. The growth arrest results in minimal shortening, if any, and is not an important complication because of the almost mature epiphysis in these patients. As for residual incongruity, it can usually be prevented by adequate reduction [34].

Ankle sprains

Ankle sprains have been reported to make up 10% to 28% of all athletic injuries [43,44]. In dealing with the younger athlete, serious ankle sprains are unusual, however, because the ligaments are usually stronger than the bone in the skeletally immature [20,21,26]. These children usually injure the distal fibular physis. More mature children or adolescents have a greater chance of a

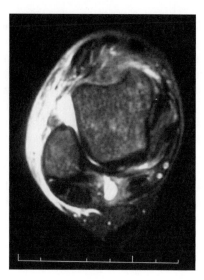

Fig. 10. MRI image of an anterior talofibular ligament (ATFL) rupture in an 11-year-old basketball player. An osteochondral lesion and distal fibular fracture were ruled out with this examination.

ligamentous injury; however, always consider a distal physeal fracture until proven otherwise (Fig. 10).

The most common mechanism of ankle sprains (as with adult athletes) is inversion and plantarflexion. Typically, this results in injury of the anterior talofibular and calcaneofibular ligaments. Careful and thorough examination of the young athlete typically demonstrates tenderness over the anterolateral ankle as opposed to the distal fibular physis. There is also overlying edema. The pain can be reproduced with an inversion stress maneuver [27,28].

Ankle sprains can be graded on a scale of I to III. Grade I sprains are the most common [28,45]. These present with pain but do not have swelling or instability. The adolescent athlete can usually return to sports in 1 to 2 weeks. Grade II sprains have marked swelling, pain, and slight laxity. These athletes usually require 8 to 12 weeks to return to their sport. Grade III sprains have gross instability, marked swelling, and, usually, severe pain. These athletes generally require some immobilization and formal rehabilitation [27,28]. The most severe sprain involves the lateral ligaments and the interosseous membrane, the so-called "high sprain." The mortise must be evaluated to ensure that there is no need for surgical correction of widening with a syndesmosis screw. If there is no radiographic instability, the athlete undergoes cast immobilization for 3 weeks, followed by intense rehabilitation [28]. Grade III and interosseous membrane injuries are more prone to chronic instability and osteochondral fractures, which may require surgical correction [27,45].

Medial ankle sprains are less common and have a higher incidence of associated syndesmosis sprains. These seem to be less stable and are treated with non–weight- bearing casting for 2 to 3 weeks, followed by rehabilitation [46].

The management of most sprains of the ankle should be conservative for at least 6 months before operative intervention is considered [27]. Athletes with recurrent sprains and no underlying problem should be treated initially with aggressive rehabilitation to strengthen peroneal musculature and proprioception. Bracing also plays a role in treatment [28,47]. Chronic problems after ankle sprains usually fall into three categories: instability, impingement, and articular lesions [48]. In recalcitrant cases, ligament reconstruction is performed, but reconstructions that require tunneling should not be performed in children with open physis [49]. A modified Broström procedure can be used in children and young adolescents [50,51]. The Broström-Gould procedure is an anatomic reconstruction of the ATFL using the inferior peroneal retinaculum to augment the construct. Results of this lateral ankle stabilization procedure have been uniformly excellent [28,52].

Acute metatarsal fractures

Metatarsal fractures are common in children participating in sports [26]. They usually occur indirectly as a result of torsional forces and avulsions or from direct trauma [53]. The fifth metatarsal is the most commonly fractured metatarsal in children (45% of all pediatric metatarsal fractures) with 90% of these fractures occurring in children less than 10 years of age (see Fig. 5; Fig. 11). Knowledge of the anatomy here is important. The fifth metatarsal has its epiphysis located distally and its apophysis located proximally. The normal apophysis is diagonal in nature, parallel to the long axis of the metatarsal, aiding in its distinction from a fracture (see discussion of Iselin's disease) [27]. An inversion stress can cause the peroneus brevis tendon to avulse the base of the metatarsal, resulting in a transverse fracture [27]. A second proposed mechanism of injury was proposed by Giachino, who believed it was secondary to the tendinous portion of the abductor digiti minimi and the lateral cord of the aponeurosis [54]. This is usually treated with a short-leg walking cast for 3 to 6 weeks [27,28].

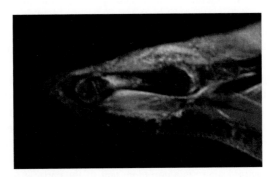

Fig. 11. MRI image of the subject in Fig. 5, confirming a fifth metatarsal shaft fracture.

Intra-articular avulsion fractures are usually transverse and are related to a traction injury from the peroneus brevis. They can be treated nonsurgically if there is minimal displacement. If there is a greater than 2- to 3-mm gap on plain radiographs, open reduction and internal fixation should be considered [28].

A fifth metatarsal fracture that occurs at the junction of the metaphysis and diaphysis is called a Jones fracture. This is less common in the skeletally immature athlete. The average age of occurrence is 15 to 21 years, and the subjects are usually involved in athletics [27]. These fractures are extremely difficult to treat secondary to the potential for delayed healing and the high complication rate. It is essential to recognize the difference between these difficult fractures and those that can simply be treated with immobilization. We recommend aggressive treatment with open reduction and internal fixation. DeLee and colleagues [55] successfully treated these fractures in young athletes with internal fixation.

Foot sprains

Turf toe

Turf toe is a first metatarsophalangeal (plantar capsule–ligament) sprain. In a more severe injury, the capsule can actually tear off the metatarsal head. There is an increasing incidence in young athletes playing on synthetic surfaces and using lighter and more flexible shoes. The injury is more common in football players but can also be seen in those who play soccer and basketball. The usual mechanism of a turf toe is hyperextension, and most of these injuries occur on artificial turf. Hyperflexion can be another mechanism, however [56].

Care should be taken to evaluate the medial and lateral collateral ligaments in addition to the position and alignment of the sesamoid bones so as to rule out concomitant injury. Plain radiographs are of marginal benefit, except to evaluate the position of the sesamoid bones. MRI is a useful modality and can identify the degree of injury in addition to identifying chondral injuries (Fig. 12).

Treatment of turf toe includes rest, ice, compression, and elevation; early joint mobilization; taping during activity; and increasing the rigidity of the shoe with a forefoot steel plate. A grade I sprain is a stretch or minor tearing of the capsuloligamentous complex with localized plantar tenderness, minimal swelling, no ecchymosis, and minimal loss of motion. The adolescent is usually able to continue playing with the toe taped. A grade II sprain is a partial tear with more tenderness, moderate swelling, and moderate ecchymosis. There is mild or moderate loss of motion and a mild limp, and symptoms worsen over 24 hours. The adolescent athlete usually cannot perform at the normal level. The athlete's playing is typically restricted for 3 to 14 days. Treatment involves immobilization in a postoperative shoe for 2 weeks.

In a grade III sprain, there is a complete tear of the capsule off the metatarsal head, severe pain plantarly and dorsally, severe swelling and ecchymosis, no

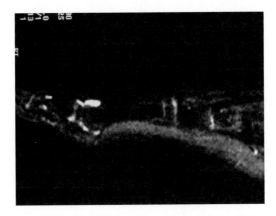

Fig. 12. MRI image of a 13-year-old female ballet dancer with a hyperflexion injury to first MTPJ. Rest and physical therapy were required to return her to dancing.

motion, and no ability to weight bear medially. A radiograph should be taken to rule out an associated sesamoid fracture [57]. Subjects with a grade III injury should use crutches for 1 to 3 days and not play for 2 to 6 weeks. In these more severe grades of ligamentous laxity, a cast is preferred, with the toe in 10° of plantarflexion to take the resting tension off the plantar structures. Return to play is indicated when the toe can be dorsiflexed 90° and then taped [57]. Surgery is restricted to recalcitrant cases and to those cases with osteochondral injury.

In general, turf toe has a less than excellent outcome, with most series reporting just more than half of patients being satisfied with the outcome [58]. Long-term results include decreased first metatarsophalangeal joint motion, impaired push off, and hallux rigidus [56]. Fifty percent of athletes have persistent symptoms 5 years later [58].

Returning the youth athlete to activity

This is, arguably, one of the most important aspects of care, which may have major implications for near-term function and future athletic potential. Although the literature is not replete with sport-specific guidelines, some general principles can be articulated in the absence of a significant body of scientific studies.

McFarland [59] identifies four factors worthy of consideration in dealing with this critically important issue. The first is the medical component and the one that is least well defined. There are significant knowledge deficits even in the most current sports medicine literature. We acquire information on a frequent basis, which may aid our decision- making process, yet there is never complete certainty, given the number and complexity of circumstances that are unique to any given athlete. The second variable is the social and/or economic factor [59]. Parental, peer, or coach pressure to return to play may be obvious or more subtle.

High-school athletes who have scholarship opportunities may feel tremendous pressure to compete even when their healing and readiness are incomplete.

McFarland [59] identifies political concerns as the third factor regarding return to play. Simply put, a clear system and chain of command regarding the physician, coach, trainer, and parents should be established, such that all acknowledge who the decision makers are under given circumstances. Thus, significant stress can be avoided in working through this process.

The final factor to consider regarding return to play is the legal issue [59]. Ultimately, the physician is obligated to put the interest of the patient first and not to bow to pressure from parents or coaches. Along the same line, medications, such as narcotics, should not be used to allow early return to play in the setting of an athlete who would otherwise be unfit or incompletely recovered.

Taylor-Butler and Landry [60] have identified general principles to be followed in considering return to play, which may be referenced regardless of the site of injury:

1. Injured joints should exhibit full range of motion without significant pain
2. Normal strength with a side-to-side differential less than 10% to 15%
3. Normal neurologic examination
4. Absence of persistent swelling
5. Absence of joint instability
6. Ability to run without pain, limping, or favoring the injured extremity (without pain medication)
7. An understanding of the need for proper warm-up and the use of taping and/or bracing to prevent reinjury when indicated
8. Comprehension of the risk of reinjury and disability

Summary

Care of the youth athlete requires knowledge of developmental anatomy and specific injury patterns, which are acute or chronic in nature. We may expect that the incidence of overuse and acute foot and ankle injuries in this population is likely to increase in proportion to the number and intensity of competitive youth teams with demanding training schedules. We, as physicians, must exercise our best judgment in regard to recognizing these patterns early and instituting appropriate treatments. Return to play decisions should be based on objective criteria when available and always keeping the best interest of the athlete's future health in the forefront of our minds.

References

[1] Wilder RT, Berde CB, Wolohan M, et al. RSDS in children. J Bone Joint Surg Am 1992;74(6): 910–9.

[2] Herring SA, Nilson KL. Introduction to overuse injuries. Clin Sports Med 1987;6:225–39.

[3] Outerbridge AR, Micheli LJ. Overuse injuries in the young athlete. Clin Sports Med 1995;14(3): 503–16.

[4] Micheli LJ. Overuse injuries in children's sports: the growth factor. Orthop Clin North Am 1983;14:337–60.

[5] Resnick DR. Osteochondroses. In: Resnick DR, editor. Diagnosis of bone and joint disorders. 4th edition. Philadelphia: WB Saunders; 2002. p. 3686–741.

[6] Sever JW. Apophysitis of the os calcis. NY J Med 1912;95:1025–9.

[7] Micheli LJ. Prevention and management of calcaneal apophysitis in children: an overuse syndrome. J Pediatr Orthop 1987;7:34–8.

[8] Gerbino PG, Micheli LJ. The lower extremity. Pediatric foot and ankle injuries. In: Scuderi GR, McCann PD, editors. Sports medicine: a comprehensive approach. Philadelphia: Elsevier Mosby; 2005. p. 485–6.

[9] Ippolito E, Ricciardi-Pollini PT, Faley F. Kohler's disease of the tarsal navicular: long-term follow-up of 12 cases. J Pediatr Orthop 1984;4(4):416–7.

[10] Chambers HG. Ankle and foot disorders in skeletally immature athletes. Orthop Clin North Am 2003;34:445–59.

[11] Williams GA, Cowell HR. Kohler's disease of the tarsal navicular. Clin Orthop 1981;158: 53–8.

[12] Schwartz B, Jay RM, Schoenhaus HD. Apophysitis of the fifth metatarsal base. Iselin's disease. J Am Podiatr Med Assoc 1991;81:128–30.

[13] Simons SM, Sloan BK. Foot injuries. In: Birrer RB, Griesemer BA, Cataletto MB, editors. Pediatric sports medicine for primary care. Philadelphia: Williams & Wilkins; 2002. p. 431–54.

[14] Griffin LY. Common sports injuries of the foot and ankle seen in children and adolescents. Orthop Clin North Am 1994;25:83–93.

[15] Hamilton W. Foot and ankle injuries and dancers. Clin Sports Med 1988;7(1):143–73.

[16] Khumbare DA. The pediatric athlete. In: Livingstone Kumbhare DA, Basmajian JV, editors. Decision making and outcomes in sports rehabilitation. New York: Churchill Livingstone; 2000. p. 223–40.

[17] Bennell KL, Brukner PD. Epidemiology and site specificity of stress fractures. Clin Sports Med 1997;16:179–96.

[18] Khan KM, Fuller PJ, Brukner PD. Outcome of conservative and surgical management of navicular stress fracture and athletes. Am J Sports Med 1992;20:657–66.

[19] Salter R, Harris W. Injuries involving the epiphyseal plate. J Bone Joint Surg Am 1963;45: 587–622.

[20] Dias LS. Fractures of the distal tibial and fibular physis. In: Rockwood Jr CA, Wilkins KE, King RE, editors. Fractures in children. 3rd edition. Philadelphia: Lippincott; 1991. p. 1314–81.

[21] McManama Jr GB. Ankle injuries in the young athlete. Clin Sports Med 1988;7:547–62.

[22] Rogers L, Poznanski A. Imaging of epiphyseal injuries. Radiology 1994;191:297–308.

[23] Dias L, Tachdjian M. Physeal injuries of the ankle in children. Clin Orthop 1978;136:230–3.

[24] Kleiger B, Mankin H. Fracture of the lateral portion of the distal tibial epiphysis. J Bone Joint Surg Am 1964;46:25–32.

[25] Landin L, Danielsson L. Children's ankle fractures. Acta Orthop Scand 1983;54:634–40.

[26] Hunter-Griffin LY. Injuries to the leg, ankle, and foot. In: Sullivan JA, Grana WA, editors. The pediatric athlete. Park Ridge (IL): American Academy of Orthopaedic Surgeons; 1990. p. 187–98.

[27] Omey ML, Micheli LJ. Foot and ankle problems in the young athlete. Med Sci Sports Exerc 1999;31(7 Suppl):S470–86.

[28] Chambers HG. Ankle and foot disorders in skeletally immature athletes. Orthop Clin North Am 2003;34:445–59.

[29] Goldberg VM, Aadalen R. Distal tibial epiphyseal injuries: the role of athletics in 3 cases. Am J Sports Med 1978;6:263–8.

[30] Cooperman D, Spiegel P, Laros G. Tibial fractures involving the ankle in children. J Bone and Joint Surg Am 1978;60:1040–6.

[31] Marmor L. The triplane distal tibial epiphyseal involving the ankle in children. J Bone Joint Surg Am 1978;60:1040–6.

[32] Lynn M. The triplane distal epiphyseal fracture. Clin Orthop 1972;86:187–90.

[33] Torg J, Ruggiero R. Comminuted epiphyseal fracture of the distal tibia. A case report and review of the literature. Clin Orthop 1975;110:215–7.

[34] Peiro A, Aracil J, Martos F, et al. Triplane distal tibial epiphyseal fracture. Clin Orthop 1981;160: 196–200.

[35] Karrholm J, Hansson L, Laurin S. Computed tomography of intraarticular supination-eversion fractures of the ankle in adolescents. J Pediatr Orthop 1981;1(2):181–7.

[36] Denton J, Fischer S. The medial triplane fracture. J Trauma 1981;21:991–5.

[37] Izant T, Davidson R. The four part triplane fracture. Foot Ankle 1989;10(3):170–5.

[38] Dias L, Giegerich C. Fractures of the distal tibial epiphysis in adolescence. J Bone Joint Surg Am 1983;65:438–44.

[39] Spiegel P, Mast J, Cooperman D, et al. Triplane fractures of the distal tibial epiphysis. Clin Orthop 1984;188:74–89.

[40] Oh W, Craig C, Bank H. Epiphyseal injuries. Pediatr Clin North Am 1974;21(2):401–22.

[41] Cone R, Nygayen V, Flournoy J, et al. Triplane fracture of the distal tibial epiphysis. Radiology 1984;153:763–7.

[42] Kornblatt N, Neese DJ, Azzolini TJ. Triplane fracture of the distal tibia: unusual case presentation and literature review. J Foot Surg 1990;29:421–8.

[43] Kaeding CC, Whithead R. Musculoskeletal injuries in adolescents. Primary Care Clin Office Pract 1998;25:211–23.

[44] Barker HB, Beynnon BD, Renstrom P. Ankle injury risk factors in sports. Sports Med 1997; 23:69–74.

[45] Wilkerson LA. Ankle injuries in athletes. Primary Care Clin Office Pract 1992;19:377–92.

[46] Tucker AM. Common soccer injuries. Sports Med 1997;23:21–32.

[47] Kennedy JG, Knowles B, Dolan M, et al. Foot and ankle injuries in the adolescent runner. Curr Opin Pediatr 2005;7:34–43.

[48] Olgilvie-Harris DJ, Gilbart MK, Chorney K. Chronic pain following ankle sprains in athletes: the role of arthroscopic surgery. Arthroscopy 1997;13:564–74.

[49] Chrisman OD, Snook GA. Reconstruction of lateral ligament tears of the ankle: an experimental study and clinical evaluation of 7 patients treated by a new modification of the Elmslie Procedure. J Bone Joint Surg Am 1969;52:904–12.

[50] Brostrom L. Sprained ankles: VI. Surgical treatment of "chronic" ligament ruptures. Acta Chir Scand 1966;132:552–65.

[51] Gould N, Selingson D, Gassman J. Early and late repair of lateral ankle ligaments of the ankle. Foot Ankle 1980;1:84–9.

[52] Robinson DE, Winson IG, Harries WJ, et al. Arthroscopic treatment of osteochondral lesions of the talus. J Bone Joint Surg Br 2003;85:989–93.

[53] Owen RJT, Hickey FG, Finlay DB. A study of metatarsal fractures in children. Injury 1995;26: 537–8.

[54] Richli WR, Rosenthal DI. Avulsion fracture of the fifth metatarsal: experimental study of pathomechanics. AJR Am J Roentgenol 1984;143(4):889–91.

[55] DeLee JC, Evans JP, Julian J. Stress fracture of the fifth metatarsal. Am J Sports Med 1983; 11:349–53.

[56] Rodeo SA, O'Brien S, Warren RF, et al. Turf toe: an analysis of metatarsophalangeal joint sprains in professional football players. Am J Sports Med 1990;18:280–5.

[57] Clanton TO, Ford JJ. Turf toe injury. Clin Sports Med 1994;13:731–41.

[58] Clanton TO, Butler JE, Eggert A. Injury to the metatarsal phalangeal joints in athletes. J Foot Ankle 1986;7:162–8.

[59] McFarland EG, editor. Preface. Clin Sports Med 2004;23(3):xv–xxiii.

[60] Taylor-Butler KL, Landry GL. Principles of healing and rehabilitation. In: Birrer RB, Greisemer BA, Cataletto MB, editors. Pediatric sports medicine for primary care. Philadelphia: Williams & Wilkins; 2002. p. 235–49.

Further readings

Gips S, Ruchman RB, Groshar D. Bone imaging in Kohler's disease. Clin Nucl Med 1997;22:636–7.

Heidt RS, Sweeterman LM, Carlonas RL, et al. Avoidance of soccer injuries with preseason conditioning. Am J Sports Med 2000;28:659–62.

Junge A, Rosch D. Prevention of soccer injuries: a prospective intervention study in youth amateur players. Am J Sports Med 2002;30:652–9.

Mann RA, Coughlin MJ, editors. Surgery of the foot and ankle, vol. 2. St. Louis (MO): Mosby–Year Book 1993. p. 1028.

Merrick MA. Secondary injury after musculoskeletal trauma: a review and update. Journal of Athletic Training 2002;37(2):209–17.

Micheli LJ, Glassman R, Klein M. The prevention of sports injuries in children. Clin Sports Med 2000;19(4):821–34.

Morgan RC. Surgical management of tarsal coalition. Foot Ankle1986;7(3):183–93.

Pappas AM. The osteochondroses. Pediatr Clin North Am 1967;14:549–70.

Putukian M. Return to play: making the tough decisions. Phys Sports Med 1998;26:25–7.

Rosen P, Micheli L, Treves S. Early scintigraphic evidence of bone stress fractures in athletic adolescents. Pediatrics 1982;70:11–5.

ELSEVIER
SAUNDERS

Clin Podiatr Med Surg
23 (2006) 233–239

CLINICS IN
PODIATRIC
MEDICINE AND
SURGERY

Index

Note: Page numbers of article titles are in **boldface** type.

Changing Your Address?

Make sure your subscription changes too! When you notify us of your new address, you can help make our job easier by including an exact copy of your Clinics label number with your old address (see illustration below.) This number identifies you to our computer system and will speed the processing of your address change. Please be sure this label number accompanies your old address and your corrected address—you can send an old Clinics label with your number on it or just copy it exactly and send it to the address listed below.

We appreciate your help in our attempt to give you continuous coverage. Thank you.

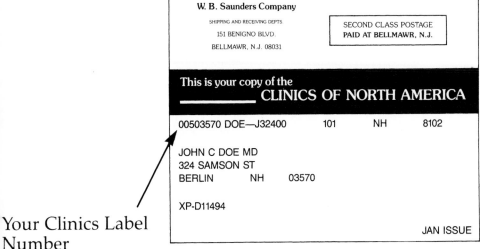

W. B. Saunders Company

SHIPPING AND RECEIVING DEPTS.
151 BENIGNO BLVD.
BELLMAWR, N.J. 08031

SECOND CLASS POSTAGE
PAID AT BELLMAWR, N.J.

This is your copy of the
_____ CLINICS OF NORTH AMERICA

00503570 DOE—J32400   101   NH   8102

JOHN C DOE MD
324 SAMSON ST
BERLIN   NH   03570

XP-D11494

JAN ISSUE

Your Clinics Label
Number
Copy it exactly or send your label
along with your address to:
W.B. Saunders Company, Customer Service
Orlando, FL 32887-4800
Call Toll Free 1-800-654-2452

Please allow four to six weeks for delivery of new subscriptions and for processing address changes.